# Coronary Risk Factors Update

*Guest Editors*

VALENTIN FUSTER, MD, PhD
JAGAT NARULA, MD, PhD

# MEDICAL CLINICS
# OF NORTH AMERICA

www.medical.theclinics.com

January 2012 • Volume 96 • Number 1

SAUNDERS an imprint of ELSEVIER, Inc.

**W.B. SAUNDERS COMPANY**
*A Division of Elsevier Inc.*

1600 John F. Kennedy Boulevard ● Suite 1800 ● Philadelphia, Pennsylvania 19103-2899

http://www.theclinics.com

**MEDICAL CLINICS OF NORTH AMERICA Volume 96, Number 1**
**January 2012 ISSN 0025-7125, ISBN-13: 978-1-4557-3889-2**

Editor: Rachel Glover
Developmental Editor: Teia Stone

*Medical Clinics of North America* (ISSN 0025-7125) is published bimonthly by Elsevier Inc., 360 Park Avenue South, New York, NY 10010-1710. Months of issue are January, March, May, July, September, and November. Periodicals postage paid at New York, NY, and additional mailing offices. Subscription prices are USD 232 per year for US individuals, USD 424 per year for US institutions, USD 117 per year for US students, USD 295 per year for Canadian individuals, USD 551 per year for Canadian institutions, USD 184 per year for Canadian students, USD 358 per year for international individuals, USD 551 per year for international institutions and USD 184 per year for international students. To receive student/resident rate, orders must be accompanied by name of affiliated institution, date of term, and the *signature* of program/residency coordinator on institution letterhead. Orders will be billed at individual rate until proof of status is received. Foreign air speed delivery is included in all *Clinics* subscription prices. All prices are subject to change without notice. **POSTMASTER:** Send address changes to *Medical Clinics of North America*, Elsevier Health Sciences Division, Subscription Customer Service, 3251 Riverport Lane, Maryland Heights, MO 63043. **Customer Service: Telephone: 1-800-654-2452** (U.S. and Canada); **1-314-447-8871** (outside U.S. and Canada). **Fax: 1-314-447-8029. E-mail: journalscustomerservice-usa@elsevier.com** (for print support); **journalsonlinesupport-usa@ elsevier.com** (for online support).

*Reprints.* For copies of 100 or more of articles in this publication, please contact the Commercial Reprints Department, Elsevier Inc., 360 Park Avenue South, New York, NY 10010-1710. Tel.: 212-633-3812; Fax: 212-462-1935; E-mail: reprints@elsevier.com.

*Medical Clinics of North America* is also published in Spanish by McGraw-Hill Interamericana Editores S. A., P.O. Box 5-237, 06500 Mexico, D.F., Mexico.

*Medical Clinics of North America* is covered in *MEDLINE/PubMed (Index Medicus), Current Contents, ASCA, Excerpta Medica, Science Citation Index,* and *ISI/BIOMED.*

Printed and bound by CPI Group (UK) Ltd, Croydon, CR0 4YY

Transferred to Digital Print 2012

## GOAL STATEMENT

The goal of *Medical Clinics of North America* is to keep practicing physicians up to date with current clinical practice by providing timely articles reviewing the state of the art in patient care.

## ACCREDITATION

The *Medical Clinics of North America* is planned and implemented in accordance with the Essential Areas and Policies of the Accreditation Council for Continuing Medical Education (ACCME) through the joint sponsorship of the University of Virginia School of Medicine and Elsevier. The University of Virginia School of Medicine is accredited by the ACCME to provide continuing medical education for physicians.

The University of Virginia School of Medicine designates this enduring material activity for a maximum of 15 *AMA PRA Category 1 Credit*(s)™ for each issue, 90 credits per year. Physicians should only claim credit commensurate with the extent of their participation in the activity.

The American Medical Association has determined that physicians not licensed in the US who participate in this CME enduring material activity are eligible for a maximum of 15 *AMA PRA Category 1 Credit*(s)™ for each issue, 90 credits per year.

Credit can be earned by reading the text material, taking the CME examination online at http://www.theclinics.com/home/cme, and completing the evaluation. After taking the test, you will be required to review any and all incorrect answers. Following completion of the test and evaluation, your credit will be awarded and you may print your certificate.

## FACULTY DISCLOSURE/CONFLICT OF INTEREST

The University of Virginia School of Medicine, as an ACCME accredited provider, endorses and strives to comply with the Accreditation Council for Continuing Medical Education (ACCME) Standards of Commercial Support, Commonwealth of Virginia statutes, University of Virginia policies and procedures, and associated federal and private regulations and guidelines on the need for disclosure and monitoring of proprietary and financial interests that may affect the scientific integrity and balance of content delivered in continuing medical education activities under our auspices.

The University of Virginia School of Medicine requires that all CME activities accredited through this institution be developed independently and be scientifically rigorous, balanced and objective in the presentation/discussion of its content, theories and practices.

All authors/editors participating in an accredited CME activity are expected to disclose to the readers relevant financial relationships with commercial entities occurring within the past 12 months (such as grants or research support, employee, consultant, stock holder, member of speakers bureau, etc.). The University of Virginia School of Medicine will employ appropriate mechanisms to resolve potential conflicts of interest to maintain the standards of fair and balanced education to the reader. Questions about specific strategies can be directed to the Office of Continuing Medical Education, University of Virginia School of Medicine, Charlottesville, Virginia.

The faculty and staff of the University of Virginia Office of Continuing Medical Education have no financial affiliations to disclose.

**The authors/editors listed below have identified no professional or financial affiliations for themselves or their spouse/partner:**

Eloisa Arbustini, MD, PhD; Juan Jose Badimon, PhD; Ragavendra R. Baliga, MD, MBA; Ailin Barseghian, MD; Roger S. Blumenthal, MD; Sonny Dandona, MD, FRCPC; Sarah D. de Ferranti, MD, MPH; Ravi Dhingra, MD, MPH; Valentin Fuster, MD, PhD (Guest Editor); Rachel Glover, (Acquisitions Editor); Nezam Haider, PhD; Randolph Hutter, MD; Payal Kohli, MD; Donald M. Lloyd-Jones, MD, ScM; Seth S. Martin, MD; Dilbahar S. Mohar, MD; Jagat Narula, MD, PhD (Guest Editor); Nupoor Narula, BS; Claudio Rapezzi, MD, FESC; William F. Rayburn, MD, MBA (Consulting Editor); Robert Roberts, MD, FRCPC, MACC; Leslee J. Shaw, PhD; Alexandre F.R. Stewart, BSch, MSc, PhD; Ramachandran S. Vasan, MD, DM; John T. Wilkins, MD, MS; Andrew Wolf, MD (Test Author).

**The authors/editors listed below identified the following professional or financial affiliations for themselves or their spouse/partner:**

**Christopher P. Cannon, MD** is an industry funded research/investigator for Accumetrics, AstraZeneca, GlaxoSmithKline, Merck, Essentialis, and Takeda, and is a consultant for Bristol-Myers Squibb/Sanofi, Novartis, and Alnylam.

**Michael Domanski, MD** is a consultant for Cardiomems.

**Yonghong Li, PhD** is employed by Celera, and is a patent holder for Quest Diagnostics.

**Michael Miller, MD** is an industry funded research/investigator and is on the Speakers' Bureau for Abbott, Merck, and Roche; is on the Advisory Committee for Abbott and Roche; and is a consultant for Roche.

**Kathryn M. Momary, PharmD, BCPS** is an industry funded research/investigator for Pfizer, Inc.

**H. Robert Superko, MD** is employed by Celera, Inc.

**Luigi Tavazzi, MD, PhD** is on the Advisory Board for Servier, Medtronic DSMB, St. Jude, and Cardiokine.

## *Disclosure of Discussion of Non-FDA Approved Uses for Pharmaceutical Products and/or Medical Devices.*

The University of Virginia School of Medicine, as an ACCME provider, requires that all faculty presenters identify and disclose any off-label uses for pharmaceutical and medical device products. The University of Virginia School of Medicine recommends that each physician fully review all the available data on new products or procedures prior to clinical use.

## TO ENROLL

To enroll in the Medical Clinics of North America Continuing Medical Education program, call customer service at 1-800-654-2452 or visit us online at http://www.theclinics.com/home/cme. The CME program is available to subscribers for an additional fee of USD 228.

FORTHCOMING ISSUES

*March 2012*
**Thyroid Disorders and Diseases**
Kenneth D. Burman, MD, *Guest Editor*

*May 2012*
**COPD**
Stephen I. Rennard, MD, and
Bartolome R. Celli, MD, *Guest Editors*

*July 2012*
**Immunotherapeutics in Clinical Medicine**
Nancy Khardori, MD, PhD, and
Romesh Khardori, MD, PhD, *Guest Editors*

RECENT ISSUES

*November 2011*
**Pulmonary Diseases**
Ali I. Musani, MD, *Guest Editor*

*September 2011*
**Obesity**
Derek LeRoith, MD, PhD, and
Eddy Karnieli, MD, *Guest Editors*

*July 2011*
**Antibacterial Therapy and Newer Agents**
Keith S. Kaye, MD, MPH, and
Donald Kaye, MD, *Guest Editors*

---

**RELATED INTEREST**

*Cardiology Clinics*, February 2011 (Volume 29, Issue 1)
**Prevention of Cardiovascular Disease: A Continuum**
Prakash Deedwania, MD, *Guest Editor*

---

**VISIT US ONLINE!**
Access your subscription at:
**www.theclinics.com**

# Contributors

## GUEST EDITORS

**VALENTIN FUSTER, MD, PhD**
Mount Sinai School of Medicine, New York, New York; Fundación Centro Nacional de Investigaciones Cardiovasculares Carlos III, Madrid, Spain

**JAGAT NARULA, MD, PhD, FACC**
Division of Cardiology, University of California-Irvine School of Medicine, Orange, California; Mount Sinai School of Medicine, New York, New York

## AUTHORS

**ELOISA ARBUSTINI, MD, PhD**
Professor, Center for Inherited Cardiovascular Diseases, Fondazione IRCCS Policlinico San Matteo, Pavia, Italy

**JUAN JOSE BADIMON, PhD**
Professor of Medicine and Director, Atherothrombosis Research Unit, Mount Sinai School of Medicine, New York, New York

**RAGAVENDRA R. BALIGA, MD, MBA**
Vice-Chief and Assistant Division Director, Division of Cardiovascular Medicine; Professor of Internal Medicine, The Ohio State University, Columbus, Ohio

**AILIN BARSEGHIAN, MD**
Division of Cardiology, University of California-Irvine School of Medicine, Orange, California; Mount Sinai School of Medicine, New York, New York

**ROGER S. BLUMENTHAL, MD**
Division of Cardiology, Department of Medicine, Johns Hopkins Ciccarone Center for the Prevention of Heart Disease, Baltimore, Maryland

**CHRISTOPHER P. CANNON, MD**
Professor of Medicine, Harvard Medical School, TIMI Study Group, Cardiovascular Division, Department of Medicine, Brigham and Women's Hospital, Boston, Massachusetts

**SONNY DANDONA, MD, FRCPC**
Assistant Professor of Medicine, Faculty of Medicine, McGill University, Montreal, Quebec, Canada

**SARAH D. DE FERRANTI, MD, MPH**
Director, Preventive Cardiology, Assistant Professor, Department of Cardiology, Children's Hospital Boston, Harvard University School of Medicine, Boston, Massachusetts

**RAVI DHINGRA, MD, MPH**
Instructor of Medicine, Section of Cardiology, Dartmouth Medical School, Heart and Vascular Center, Dartmouth-Hitchcock Medical Center, Lebanon, New Hampshire

**MICHAEL DOMANSKI, MD**
Division of Cardiology, University of California-Irvine School of Medicine, Orange, California; Mount Sinai School of Medicine, New York, New York

**VALENTIN FUSTER, MD, PhD**
Mount Sinai School of Medicine, New York, New York; Fundación Centro Nacional de Investigaciones Cardiovasculares Carlos III, Madrid, Spain

**NEZAM HAIDER, PhD**
Division of Cardiology, University of California-Irvine School of Medicine, Orange, California; Mount Sinai School of Medicine, New York, New York

**RANDOLPH HUTTER, MD**
Research Fellow in Cardiology, Mount Sinai School of Medicine, New York, New York

**PAYAL KOHLI, MD**
Fellow, TIMI Study Group, Cardiovascular Division, Department of Medicine, Brigham and Women's Hospital, Boston, Massachusetts

**YONGHONG LI, PhD**
Principal Scientist, Celera Corporation, Alameda, California

**DONALD M. LLOYD-JONES, MD, ScM**
Departments of Preventive Medicine and Medicine, Northwestern University Feinberg School of Medicine, Chicago, Illinois

**SETH S. MARTIN, MD**
Division of Cardiology, Department of Medicine, Johns Hopkins Ciccarone Center for the Prevention of Heart Disease, Baltimore, Maryland

**MICHAEL MILLER, MD**
Division of Cardiology, Department of Medicine, Center for Preventive Cardiology, University of Maryland Medical Center, Baltimore, Maryland

**DILBAHAR S. MOHAR, MD**
Division of Cardiology, University of California-Irvine School of Medicine, Orange, California; Mount Sinai School of Medicine, New York, New York

**KATHRYN M. MOMARY, PharmD, BCPS**
Assistant Professor, Mercer University College of Pharmacy and Health Sciences, Atlanta, Georgia

**JAGAT NARULA, MD, PhD, FACC**
Division of Cardiology, University of California-Irvine School of Medicine, Orange, California; Mount Sinai School of Medicine, New York, New York

**NUPOOR NARULA, BS**
Center for Inherited Cardiovascular Diseases, Fondazione IRCCS Policlinico San Matteo, Pavia, Italy

**CLAUDIO RAPEZZI, MD**
Institute of Cardiology, University of Bologna and Policlinico S. Orsola-Malpighi Hospital, Bologna, Italy

**ROBERT ROBERTS, MD, FRCPC, MACC**
Professor of Medicine and Director, Ruddy Canadian Cardiovascular Genetics Centre; President and CEO, University of Ottawa Heart Institute, Ottawa, Ontario, Canada

**LESLEE J. SHAW, PhD**
Professor of Medicine and Co-Director, Emory Clinical Cardiovascular Research Institute, Emory University School of Medicine, Atlanta, Georgia

**ALEXANDRE F.R. STEWART, BSch, MSc, PhD**
Principal Investigator, Ruddy Canadian Cardiovascular Genetics Centre, Ottawa, Ontario, Canada

**H. ROBERT SUPERKO, MD, FACC, FAHA, FAACVPR**
Chief Medical Officer, Celera Corporation, Alameda, California; Clinical Professor, Mercer University College of Pharmacy and Health Sciences; Saint Joseph's Hospital of Atlanta, Atlanta, Georgia

**LUIGI TAVAZZI, MD**
Professor, Direzione Scientifica, GVM Care and Research, Presso Maria Cecilia Hospital, Cotignola, Italy

**RAMACHANDRAN S. VASAN, MD, DM, FACC, FAHA**
Professor of Medicine and Chief, Section of Preventive Medicine and Epidemiology, Department of Medicine, Boston University School of Medicine, Boston; Framingham Heart Study, Framingham, Massachusetts

**JOHN T. WILKINS, MD, MS**
Departments of Preventive Medicine and Medicine, Northwestern University Feinberg School of Medicine, Chicago, Illinois

# Contents

therapy, residual cardiovascular risk persists and has been attributed to the persistence of atherogenic dyslipidemia and, in part, elevated triglycerides (TGs). In this review, the authors focus on the mechanism of elevated TGs and provide a discussion of the challenges of measuring TGs as a biomarker, its role in the pathogenesis of atherosclerotic heart disease, and results of several recent studies that have elucidated the relationship between TGs and cardiovascular morbidity and mortality.

In diabetes, glycation is a nonenzymatic posttranslational modification resulting from the bonding of a sugar molecule with a protein or lipid followed by oxidation, resulting in the development of advanced glycation end products (AGE). Like glycation, carbamylation is a posttranslational protein modification that is associated with AGE formation. Glycation of extracellular matrix proteins and low-density lipoprotein with subsequent deposition in the vessel wall could contribute to inflammatory response and atheroma formation. It is logical to extrapolate that carbamylation may result in modification of vessel wall proteins similar to glycation, and predispose to atherosclerosis.

This article presents an overview of clinical and molecular genetics of myocardial infarction (MI). Discussion includes the partial overlapping of risk factors for myocardial infarction and atherosclerosis, the impact of a positive family history on the risk of MI, the "familial" nongenetic, environmental factors, the inherited risk associated with the low-dose input of many genes, and a simple approach to stratify the individual risk in genetic counseling.

The risk of developing cardiovascular disease (CVD) is generally dependent on the presence or absence of traditional risk factors. Age is a well-known traditional risk factor, generally considered nonmodifiable. This review discusses the common use of individual age in prediction of CVD incidence using different risk scores, whether or not age as a risk factor can be modified, the methods used to evaluate long-term and short-term CVD risk, appropriate communication of individual risk based on age group and CVD risk, and the influence of age on cardiac and vascular risk factors.

The cardiovascular protection provided to women during the reproductive age and the unique angiogenic properties of the female reproductive system provide insights into the complex regulatory network of female sex hormones, angiogenic growth factors, and stem cell regulatory molecules. The intricate and interwoven endometrial physiology of the female menstrual cycle shows that in order to harness the physiologic cardioprotection provided by nature to women of reproductive age, for better cardiovascular therapies in postmenopausal women and the population in general, a coherent and systematic approach is needed.

Cardiovascular disease deaths have declined considerably, with more than 35% reductions during the past two decades, yet a sizable detection gap remains. Cardiovascular disease remains the leading cause of morbidity and mortality in the United States and across the world, including in developing and developed nations. Recent statistics reveal that approximately 840,000 deaths were attributed to cardiovascular disease, approximately 300,000 more deaths than reported for cancer; three-quarters were reported in previously asymptomatic individuals, raising the question as to whether screening for cardiovascular disease is warranted in detecting potentially high-risk patients.

The next decade will focus on identifying the missing heritability of coronary artery disease (CAD). This process will involve a more comprehensive interrogation of common single nucleotide polymorphisms (SNPs) that impart modest biologic effect and an interrogation of rare SNPs that impart profound biologic effect. In parallel, an investigation of the underlying biology of the described association will likely yield novel pathways that provide therapeutic targets. Once we obtain a more complete inventory of sequence variation that predisposes to CAD, a more realistic assessment of the role of genetic risk scoring allied with standard risk algorithms will be possible.

3-Hydroxy-3-methylglutaryl coenzyme A reductase inhibitor medications, commonly referred to as statins, are among the most widely prescribed medications. Variation in individual response to statins concerning low-density lipoprotein cholesterol reduction, clinical event benefit, and side effects has been observed. Some of this variability is attributed to demographic and environmental issues, chief of which is compliance. A large portion of the individual response to statin therapy is attributed to single nucleotide polymorphisms that have recently been elucidated, several of which seem to have clinical utility.

Pediatric cholesterol disorders are common, affecting 1 in 5 adolescents, although most are mild or moderate abnormalities. Because cholesterol values during childhood are moderately predictive of adult cholesterol levels, and are associated with atherosclerosis by pathology and by vascular testing, and because familial hyperlipidemias are associated with early cardiovascular events, cholesterol screening is recommended during childhood. Identified lipid abnormalities are an indication for lifestyle improvement and, in rare cases, pharmacotherapy. However, many gaps in the pediatric knowledge base remain about the benefits and risk, the optimal method for lipid screening, and about appropriate indications for pharmacotherapy.

# Preface

# Risk Factor Update: Old Wine in a New Bottle?

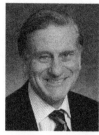 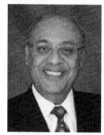

Valentin Fuster, MD, PhD     Jagat Narula, MD, PhD
*Guest Editors*

Cardiovascular diseases continue to be the leading cause of death and disability in the twenty-first century and equally affect men and women, in both developed and under-privileged nations. Most human societies have moved from agrarian diets and active lives to fast foods and sedentary habits in the last century. Combined with increasing tobacco use, these changes have fueled the epidemic of obesity, diabetes, hypertension, dyslipidemia, and cardiovascular diseases. Furthermore, while developed countries witnessed these changes over several decades due to a long period of epidemiological transition, the alterations in developing countries are occurring at an accelerated pace, calling into focus creative and innovative solutions for combating the consequences.

Coronary artery disease (CAD) was a national epidemic and the leading cause of death during 1930-1950. Although at that time CAD and acute coronary events were perceived as an inescapable consequence of old age and genetic transmission, epidemiological research, especially from the Framingham Heart Study, identified risk factors that predisposed to CAD. Risk factors were equally applicable at all ages and in either sex; there was a demonstrable causal relationship between the risk factor and the disease with a dose-response relationship to the extent of disease, and a decrease in the burden of disease on resolution of risk factors. Because the disease could be fatal even in its first manifestation and occur without warning signals even in asymptomatic subjects, a preventive approach was deemed mandatory. Immense emphasis was placed on public awareness about the risk factors, and multiple national prevention programs were initiated especially directed against hypercholesterolemia, hypertension, and smoking. More than a 50% reduction was observed in the mortality attributed to cardiovascular diseases in the latter half of the last century, a fivefold superior outcome as compared to noncardiovascular infirmity. However, a large proportion of such benefit was related to the treatment of already manifest disease rather than prevention, resulting in an enormous economic burden.

Med Clin N Am 96 (2012) xiii–xiv
doi:10.1016/j.mcna.2012.02.003
0025-7125/12/$ – see front matter

To maintain a winning streak, it has become mandatory that we emphasize cardio-vascular disease prevention and health promotion worldwide. This issue of the *Medical Clinics of North America* is dedicated to readdressing the relevance of recognizing and optimizing the risk factors. Increasingly conservative standards are being established for modifiable risk factors. It is becoming obvious that the *normal* values for risk factors (such as blood pressure and cholesterol) cannot be based on the *average* values for our populations, which are in fact the *commonly prevalent* values for the population at risk of dying from atherosclerotic disease. It is also necessary that we recognize that the burden of cardiovascular disease arises from people with cumulative load imposed by modest elevations of numerous risk factors and not with extreme elevation of a single risk factor. Further, we make an attempt to convince the readers that nonmodifiable predisposing factors may not necessarily be considered fatalistic. For instance, age may not comprise a risk factor but may represent the length of exposure to the risk factor. Similarly for family history, one may usually inherit risk factors and not vascular disease, and prevention of the risk factors should prevent disease.

It has also become mandatory that cross-continental collaboration be established, not only because the developing nations can learn tremendously from the available experience of the last century pertaining to the dynamics of risk factor upregulation and disease burden, but also the developed nations can get access to the accelerated disease pattern to learn the pathogenesis and preventive strategies better. The opportunity to study the same diseases that we witnessed 50 years ago with the modern tools and knowledge promises revolutionary information for health care in our country.

With promotion of cardiovascular health in mind, we hope that this issue of *Medical Clinics* will allow readers to look at the risk factors more aggressively and effectively. It is an extension of the age-old principles. Neither too new a wine nor too new a bottle…

Valentin Fuster, MD, PhD
Mount Sinai School of Medicine
1 Gustave L. Levy Place, Box 1030
New York, NY 10029-6574, USA

Fundación Centro Nacional de Investigaciones
Cardiovasculares Carlos III
Melchor Fernández Almagro, 3
E-28029 Madrid, Spain

Jagat Narula, MD, PhD
Mount Sinai School of Medicine
1 Gustave L. Levy Place, Box 1030
New York, NY 10029-6574, USA

E-mail addresses:
valentin.fuster@mountsinai.org (V. Fuster)
jagat.narula@mountsinai.org (J. Narula)

# Are Novel Serum Biomarkers Informative?

John T. Wilkins, MD, MS,[a,b], Donald M. Lloyd-Jones, MD, ScM[a,b],*

**KEYWORDS**

- Serum biomarkers • Coronary heart disease risk
- Risk assessment

The global burden of coronary heart disease (CHD) is massive. Fortunately, multiple lifestyle and pharmacologic therapies are available to delay the onset or progression of atherosclerosis and reduce the risk of developing clinical CHD events.[1] Myocardial infarction and myocardial infarction-related death (CHD events) are acute, discrete events that often present dramatically. The underlying disease process, however, is usually coronary artery atherosclerosis, an insidious disease process that often begins in adolescence and young adulthood and progresses over decades in most individuals.[2] The high morbidity and mortality associated with CHD events, the ability to prevent or delay these events substantially, and the high population burden of CHD make it an exceptional target for population-wide screening and prevention efforts. For acute CHD events like myocardial infarction, clinicians and health policy makers have traditionally focused on screening for the risk for disease not for the presence of disease. Thus, by its nature, assessment of risk is a probabilistic, not deterministic, exercise. This is an essential distinction from screening programs designed to detect disease in early, preclinical stages (as in cancer, for example) in an effort to reduce morbidity and mortality associated with disease.

During the past 20 years, considerable effort has been made to develop techniques for CHD risk estimation and risk stratification of asymptomatic individuals. One of the earliest techniques for risk stratification developed was the Framingham Risk Score (FRS), which predicts 10-year absolute risks for CHD events using multivariable equations containing covariates for each of the major traditional risk factors (age, gender, smoking, diabetes, total cholesterol and high-density lipoprotein cholesterol [HDL-C],

Disclosures: None.
[a] Department of Preventive Medicine, Northwestern University Feinberg School of Medicine, 680 North Lakeshore Drive, Suite 1400, Chicago, IL 60611, USA
[b] Department of Medicine, Northwestern University Feinberg School of Medicine, 251 East Huron Street, Galter Pavilion, Suite 3-150, Chicago, IL, USA
* Corresponding author. Department of Preventive Medicine, Northwestern University Feinberg School of Medicine, 680 North Lakeshore Drive, Suite 1400, Chicago, IL 60611.
*E-mail address:* dlj@northwestern.edu

and blood pressure).[3,4] This score is currently the most widely used risk estimation equation and has been incorporated into the National Cholesterol Education Program Adult Treatment Panel III (ATP III) guidelines for primary prevention.[3] ATP III suggests 3 arbitrary risk categories: low, intermediate, and high (<10%, 10%–20%, and >20%, respectively). ATP III guidelines recommend that the intensity of CHD prevention efforts (ie, the decision about whether to add pharmacologic lipid-lowering therapy to lifestyle interventions) be proportional to the risk for CHD events in the 10-year time horizon. Although useful in this population-wide screening strategy, the FRS is not perfect and essentially estimates probabilities for CHD events; thus, events still occur in individuals who are at low risk. Because of the large size of the low-risk group, a substantial proportion of CHD events still occur in this segment of the population. Therefore, in an effort to refine risk estimation and to develop a deeper understanding of the pathophysiology of CHD events, many novel serum, lipid, genetic and imaging biomarkers have been developed.

Several proposed biomarkers are significantly associated with future CHD events independent of traditional risk factors, and they provide insight into the underlying biology of CHD events. Likewise, biomarkers may assist in risk assessment in niche populations of patients, for example, people with strong family histories of premature CHD, individuals at intermediate risk for CHD events by traditional risk estimates, or individuals with unique biology (increased predilection for thrombosis or occult dyslipidemia) that may predispose to CHD events. These biomarkers, although statistically significant, typically have only modest independent associations with risk for CHD. To become a clinically useful predictor of CHD risk, a biomarker must be standardized, accurate, precise, cost effective, and reproducible in large, diverse populations. Furthermore, the novel biomarker must add predictive information over and above techniques currently in use.[5] To date, few novel biomarkers achieve this. This review includes a discussion of the specific metrics currently in use to assess the performance of biomarkers for risk prediction in the general population. These characteristics can be quantified through statistical tests that assess the calibration, discrimination, and risk reclassification capacity of biomarkers and novel risk prediction models that incorporate them.

## CALIBRATION

Calibration refers to the ability of a model to predict absolute risk accurately through comparison of predicted risk, derived from the derivation cohort, with observed risk as determined by a validation cohort. This is often done visually by dividing a population into deciles of predicted CHD risk as determined by the multivariate model and then comparing absolute observed risks with predicted risks. For a well-calibrated model, the predicted and observed event rates are similar in each stratum. The adequacy of calibration is quantified by the Hosmer-Lemeshow statistic; $P<.05$ suggests poor model calibration.

## DISCRIMINATION

The ability of a risk score (or biomarker) to discriminate CHD risk across the entire range of values is assessed by the receiver operating characteristic (ROC) curve and the area under the ROC curve (equivalent to the C statistic). The ROC curve is a plot of sensitivity versus 1-specificity (effectively, a likelihood ratio) of the risk score (**Fig. 1**). For many diagnostic tests, interrogation of this curve may be done to optimize thresholds for maximal sensitivity and/or specificity of a test, depending on the function of the particular test. Integration of the curve yields the capacity of the test to

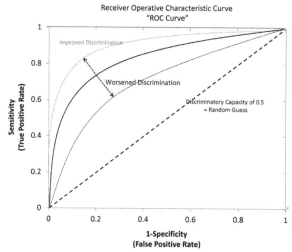

**Fig. 1.** Hypothetical receiver-operating characteristics (ROC) curve. Movement of the curve towards the upper left corner of the graph represents improved discrimination. Conversely, movement towards the line of unity represents worsened discrimination.

distinguish cases from noncases across all output values of the risk prediction model. In essence, this provides a measure of the value of the risk score or biomarker as a population-wide screening test. A C statistic value of 0.5 represents the predictive value of a coin flip, and a value of 1.0, which is unlikely to occur, is perfect discrimination. In the case of prognostic analyses, such as risk prediction, the value of the C statistic is likely dependent on the time of follow-up: noncases at one point in time may become cases with longer follow-up. For reference, the FRS model typically yields a C statistic value of 0.75 to 0.80,[6] representing excellent discrimination by contemporary standards, for future CHD events.

## NET RECLASSIFICATION IMPROVEMENT

The net reclassification improvement (NRI) quantifies the effect of a new biomarker on appropriate classification of risk when a new risk assessment algorithm stratifies individuals into categories of risk compared with an older algorithm. The NRI is generated from analysis of reclassification tables. In short, these are tables that tabulate individuals who had and did not have events and determine whether application of a novel biomarker or risk score provides significant improvement in risk classification compared with a base model. A conceptual model of the NRI is provided in **Table 1** with hypothetical risk categories. In essence, the NRI is calculated by observing the performance of the original and the modified models in individuals who did and who did not have CHD events. Among individuals who had events during the time period of observation, the number of individuals who moved down in predicted risk is subtracted from the number who appropriately moved up in predicted risk; this difference is then divided by the total number of events. The inverse operation is preformed on individuals who did not have events: the number who moved up in predicted risk is subtracted from the number who correctly moved down in predicted risk and this difference is divided by the number of individuals who did not have events. These 2 values are then summed to estimate the NRI, which has a value of −2 (perfectly

**Table 1**
Conceptual model of the net reclassification improvement (NRI)

| | | Cohort Participants With Events | | | | | Cohort Participants Without Events | | |
|---|---|---|---|---|---|---|---|---|---|
| | | Revised Model | | | | | Revised Model | | |
| | | Stratum 1 | Stratum 2 | Stratum 3[a] | | | Stratum 1 | Stratum 2 | Stratum 3[a] |
| **Original Model** | Stratum 1 | No Change | Appropriate | Appropriate | **Original Model** | Stratum 1 | No Change | Inappropriate | Inappropriate |
| | Stratum 2 | Inappropriate | No Change | Appropriate | | Stratum 2 | Appropriate | No Change | Inappropriate |
| | Stratum 3[a] | Inappropriate | Inappropriate | No Change | | Stratum 3[a] | Appropriate | Appropriate | No Change |

$$NRI = \frac{No.\ With\ Events\ Who\ Moved\ Up - No.\ With\ Events\ Who\ Moved\ Down}{Total\ No.\ With\ Events} + \frac{No.\ Without\ Events\ Who\ Moved\ Down - No.\ Without\ Events\ Who\ Moved\ Up}{Total\ No.\ Without\ Events}$$

a Table assumes ordinal strata of predicted risk with Stratum 3 as the highest risk stratum.

incorrect reclassification) to +2 (perfectly correct reclassification). To date, many novel serum biomarkers have yielded NRI values of 0.02 to 0.10.[6]

## CURRENT TECHNIQUES FOR RISK STRATIFICATION

Analysis of cohort data from the Framingham Heart Study identified several independent risk factors for CHD events. Candidate risk factors were determined by observing associations between variables at the initiation of follow-up and the subsequent development of a CHD event for approximately 10 years. The variables were then incorporated into a multivariable statistical model to assess for independence of effect on risk for CHD. The variables—age, gender, tobacco use, systolic blood pressure, need for antihypertension medication use, total cholesterol, and HDL-C—were determined to have the greatest predictive power when incorporated together in the statistical model. This model, FRS, has been validated in many different cohorts. It has been shown to discriminate 10-year risk for CHD events well across multiple race groups.[6] From a historical perspective, several of the risk factors incorporated into the model would be termed biomarkers by contemporary definitions, most notably total cholesterol, HDL-C, and systolic blood pressure.

Although the performance of the FRS statistical model is good in terms of population-wide screening performance metrics, there are some limitations to its clinical application. First, like all scientific models, there is a degree of uncertainty that must be assumed in the interpretation of the model output. Despite the most careful methodology, there is error in the measurement of all variables included in the model. For example, a one-time measurement of blood pressure may not accurately reflect usual blood pressure; error in the assessment of outcome may result in misclassification; and other sources of biologic variability may reduce the overall accuracy of the model. Thus, the results should be interpreted as an estimate of risk. Second, this estimate is derived from the behavior of the population from which it was derived and as such may reflect the factors driving the incidence of disease in the population, but it may not reflect the biology of an individual patient or completely explain the true risk for occurrence in an individual patient evaluated in a clinic.[7] It is a probability, because individuals do not have a risk of 6% for CHD; they either have CHD (100% rate) or do not have CHD (0% rate) during the period of observation. Nonetheless, all of evidence-based medicine relies on the application of efficacious strategies demonstrated in populations to individual patients with the assumption that population mean effects, on average, benefit individual patients as well. Third, as discussed previously, the discriminatory power of the model is not perfect and, the authors venture to say, never will be. Furthermore, the majority of events occur in individuals with at least one elevated risk factor but who by FRS are at low to intermediate predicted risk.[8] The fourth limitation of the FRS is that it only provides 10-year estimates of absolute risk for CHD events. The underlying disease process that predisposes most patients to CHD events, however, occurs over multiple decades, and earlier intervention in the atherosclerotic process may reduce the probability of future events. Fifth, like all multivariable equations, a relative weight related to the variance of the outcome is assigned to each variable. Not surprisingly, age has the strongest effect on CHD events and often overshadows the effect that may be attributable to other variables.

The contribution of other factors, including novel serum biomarkers, to the estimation of absolute risk could be examined in age-specific risk scores. For example, Zethelius and colleagues[9] examined the predictive value of troponin I (TnI), NT-proBNP, cystatin C, C-reactive protein (CRP), and traditional risk factors for CVD death in a cohort of 71-year-old Swedish men. By limiting their analysis to 71-year-old men they effectively removed age as a predictor variable. Using this age-specific model, they observed a significant increase in the C statistic from 0.688 to 0.748 and an NRI of 0.26 when the aforementioned serum biomarkers were added to a model with traditional risk factors. These results suggest that there may be significant room for biomarkers to explain the variance of the outcome and thus aid in risk prediction in population-wide screening if age-specific models are developed.

The biomarkers, however, that likely are relevant at one age may not be relevant for other age groups. For example, biomarkers of end-organ damage (such as TnI) may not have sufficient prevalence in younger patients to be useful population-wide predictors. Currently, insufficient age-specific cohort data are available to generate stable age-specific CHD risk estimates. Despite the limitations of FRS and other scores like it, multivariable risk scores remain the best available population-wide risk estimation tools.

## INDIVIDUAL BIOMARKERS

A detailed discussion of all novel serum biomarkers is not possible in the scope of this review. Several examples are discussed that demonstrate some key strengths and limitations of novel biomarkers. Specifically, CRP, apolipoprotein (Apo) B, lipoprotein (a) (Lp(a)), and TnI are discussed in case studies to illustrate the performance of serum biomarkers in population-wide risk assessment and the possible situations in which they may provide useful information for the clinician.

### CRP

CRP measured by current high-sensitivity assays is one of the most widely studied novel serum biomarkers. CRP is a marker of inflammation, which has been shown to have independent associations with CHD events. The biologic underpinnings of this association are likely due to chronic low-level inflammation in the vascular intima. Inflammation, however, is associated with many non-CVD disease processes; thus, elevated CRP is a nonspecific marker of cardiovascular disease.

Nevertheless, multiple community-based cohort, clinical trial, and case-control studies demonstrate robust, independent associations between elevated levels of high-sensitivity CRP and risk for CHD events. In the Physicians' Health Study, the relative risk for CHD events in individuals with CRP values greater than or equal to 2.1 mg/dL was 2.9 compared with individuals with CRP levels less than or equal to 0.55 mg/dL. Similar independent associations between elevated CRP (typically >3.0 mg/dL) and CHD events have been reproduced in multiple cohorts.[10–12] When the metrics of discrimination and NRI are applied to CRP, however, its ability to add to the discriminatory capacity of the FRS is limited. CRP did seem to have a modest effect on reclassification in individuals at intermediate risk for CHD events (10%–20% predicted 10-year risk). In a US Preventive Services Task Force–sponsored meta-analysis[13] evaluating the utility of high-sensitivity CRP for prediction of CHD events, the relative risk for incident CHD was 1.58 (95% CI, 1.37–1.83) for CRP values greater than 3.0 compared with levels less than 1.0 mg/L. CRP was found to have desirable test characteristics because it provided a modest improvement in model calibration and in reclassification of intermediate-risk individuals.[13] Thus, it may be a useful serum biomarker for the reclassification of patients at intermediate risk when decisions regarding lipid-lowering therapy remain unclear. It is less useful for those at high or low predicted risk, suggesting that it not be used as a population-wide screening tool.

Lipid lowering with rosuvastatin (20 mg) was assessed in individuals, most or whom, were at low or intermediate risk for CHD, by FRS and who had CRP greater than

2.0 mg/dL. Individuals on therapy had significant reductions in CHD events compared with placebo-treated patients, and the trial was stopped early due to significant benefit.[14] The trial did not include a low-CRP arm, however, so it is not clear if measurement of CRP specifically identifies individuals who are more likely to benefit from statin therapy.

## Apolipoprotein B

ApoB is a structural protein that exists in a 1:1 ratio with all atherogenic lipid fractions (low-density lipoprotein [LDL], very low-density lipoprotein [VLDL], and intermediate-density lipoprotein [IDL]) and likely plays a causative role in atherosclerosis development. In constitutive physiology, ApoB has an essential role in the transport of atherogenic particles from the liver to the periphery, where it is deposited in the vascular intima, thus setting the stage for retention of lipid particles, subsequent macrophage uptake, oxidation, and the eventual formation of atheroma.[15] In terms of CHD risk assessment, measurement of serum ApoB concentrations may provide some advantage compared with traditional measures of cholesterol concentration.

Measurement of ApoB has several practical advantages compared with measurement of LDL cholesterol (LDL-C). ApoB is directly measured from the serum; thus, the accuracy of the ApoB measurement is greater. Usually, LDL-C is calculated using the Friedewald equation (LDL-C = TC - HDL-C - triglycerides/5), where $TC$ is total cholesterol; the LDL-C estimate includes the error in TC, HDL, and triglyceride measurement, thus reducing its accuracy. Another advantage of the measurement of ApoB is that an estimate of atherogenic particle burden can be obtained without requiring patients to fast before the blood draw. This makes point-of-care lipid assessment logistically simpler for patients and clinicians.

ApoB is a strong predictor of future CHD events; however, in observational cohorts its predictive power is not convincingly superior to traditional lipid subfractions. In some instances these associations have been stronger than the associations observed with traditional lipid risk factors. In the Apolipoprotein Proteins Related Mortality Risk (AMORIS) study, for example, baseline ApoB concentration had an adjusted relative risk of 1.43 in men and 1.34 in women over 5 to 6 years for future CHD events. Compared with LDL-C as a predictor, ApoB had a higher sensitivity and specificity as determined by ROC curve analysis.[16] In a post hoc analysis of the Air Force/Texas Coronary Atherosclerosis Prevention Study (AFCAPS/TEXCAPS) trial, ApoB concentrations predicted future events better than LDL-C by stepwise regression analysis. ApoB also retained a stronger association with future CHD events than LDL-C for patients on lovastatin therapy. This suggests that ApoB could be an excellent target of therapy and prognostic indicator for individuals on statin therapy.[17]

Alternatively, a recent analysis from the Emerging Risk Factors Collaboration failed to demonstrate any improvement in risk prediction for ApoB compared with LDL-C.[18] A meta-analysis by Snidermann and colleagues[19] of all published studies suggests that ApoB may be superior to LDL-C and non–HDL-C as a CHD risk predictor. As is true with most novel serum biomarkers, when assessed by the rigor of calibration, discrimination, and NRI, the ApoB/ApoA1 ratio did not yield increased model performance compared with the traditional FRS when applied to the Framingham Offspring Study.[20] Thus, its use as a population-wide screening test has not been sufficiently validated.

ApoB levels, however, may also provide important information about the individual biology of patients that may potentially guide clinical decision making. Individuals with metabolic syndrome may have significantly elevated LDL particle numbers (hence, elevated ApoB) despite low to moderate LDL-C values. Increased LDL particle number and an increase in small, dense LDLs are thought to increase the atherogenicity of LDL due to enhanced diffusion of LDL into the vascular intimal space.[21] Because of the 1:1 ratio of ApoB with LDL, IDL, and VLDL particles, ApoB serves as a surrogate for LDL particle number. Thus, in patients with metabolic syndrome or diabetes, high ApoB with normal LDL may suggest occult dyslipidemia and warrant lipid-lowering therapy in patients who would otherwise be untreated. In particular, this strategy may be useful in younger patients with metabolic syndrome who may not meet clear treatment thresholds by ATP III criteria. Likewise, ApoB may be a superior target of therapy in patients with "metabolic" lipid profiles, because assessment of LDL may underestimate atherogenic lipid burden even after treatment. No trial data are available, however, to assess whether this is a clinically useful strategy.

### Lipoprotein (a)

Lp(a) is a modified LDL subtype. In brief, the Lp(a) molecule is an ApoB molecule covalently bonded to a large, hydrophilic, carbohydrate-rich moiety, known as apolipoprotein (a). The apolipoprotein (a) moiety contains multiple Kringle domains, which are believed to have biochemical homology with plasminogen. This plasminogen-like factor may alter the coagulation cascade to favor arterial thrombosis and thus increase the risks for CHD events. Multiple epidemiologic studies demonstrate significant associations between elevated Lp(a) serum concentrations (>30 mg/dL) and risk for CHD events.[22,23] A recent large meta-analysis of 36 studies, including approximately 1.3 million person years of follow-up, demonstrated independent, modest associations between elevated Lp(a) and nonfatal myocardial infarction and CHD death.[24] Lp(a) values do not correlate significantly with traditional lipid subfractions. Furthermore, observational evidence from offspring studies suggests Lp(a) is highly heritable.[25] Given the independent risks associated with Lp(a), the inability to estimate Lp(a) levels based on presence of traditional risk factors, and the strong pattern of inheritance of this molecule, some clinicians use Lp(a) in the assessment of patients with strong family histories of premature CHD. If justification for lipid-lowering therapy cannot be made on the evaluation of traditional risk factors, the presence of elevated Lp(a) can be a helpful way to unmask occult dyslipidemia and genetic risk. There are no data, however, on C statistic or NRI associated with elevated levels of Lp(a); thus, its role in population-wide screening is unclear.

### Troponin I

TnI is a myocardium-specific protein that is part of constitutive myocardial function. An elevation in TnI of greater than or equal to 2 times the upper limit of normal is used as a sensitive and specific diagnostic test to help identify myocardial injury during acute coronary syndromes. Recently, higher-sensitivity troponin assays have been developed. These highly sensitive assays may detect subclinical end-organ damage and are currently being assessed as biomarkers of increased risk for myocardial infarction, CHD death, and heart failure hospitalizations. The direct biologic connection and phenotypic similarity between subclinical TnI elevation and myocardial infarction, as well as the ease of measurement, make this an attractive biomarker for CHD risk stratification. Alternatively, it may be that waiting until subclinical myocyte damage occurs is too late in the progression of cardiovascular disease to gain maximal benefit from preventive interventions.

In a substudy analysis from the Prevention Of Events With Angiotensin Country Enzyme (PEACE) trial in patients with CHD, investigators found independent, graded associations between increases in the TnI and the risk of CHD death and incident heart failure.[26] Similar observations have been made in individuals without established CHD. An analysis conducted in the Atherosclerosis Risk in Communities Study (ARIC) [27] demonstrated independent associations between elevated TnI levels (found in approximately 65% of ARIC participants) and future CHD events, mortality, and incident heart failure. Furthermore, addition of TnI to their risk assessment model added modestly to risk prediction via improvements in the C statistic (increase of approximately 0.01–0.03) and a favorable NRI.[27] Similar associations and risk score performance have recently been reported in the Dallas Heart Study and the Cardiovascular Health Study.[28,29] In the Dallas Heart Study, elevated TnI was also associated with underlying structural heart disease. Thus, TnI may add modestly to population-wide risk stratification by inexpensively identifying occult structural heart disease or individuals with an elevated risk of heart failure.

In summary, biomarker investigation continues to give insight into the biologic mechanisms of the CVD epidemic. Patient care may be enhanced in some specific clinical scenarios by novel serum biomarkers because they can give clinicians insight into individual-level risks. In particular, serum biomarkers may be useful in patients with family history of premature CHD or patients with metabolic syndrome, in detecting patients with occult structural heart disease, or in patients at intermediate risk by ATP III criteria. Population-wide screening strategies, however, with currently available serum biomarkers are unlikely to yield substantial progress based on currently available data. Further investigation into biomarkers is necessary as is continued collection of cohort data on CHD risk. With expanded cohort data and improved biomarkers, current risk-estimation techniques to help enhance prevention strategies and reduce the population burden of CHD may, in the future, be improved.

## REFERENCES

1. Murray CJ, Lopez AD. Alternative projections of mortality and disability by cause 1990-2020: global burden of disease study. Lancet 1997;349:1498–504.
2. Natural history of aortic and coronary atherosclerotic lesions in youth. Findings from the PDAY Study. Pathobiological Determinants of Atherosclerosis in Youth (PDAY) Research Group. Arterioscler Thromb 1993;13(9):1291–8.
3. National Cholesterol Education Program (NCEP) Expert Panel on Detection, Evaluation, and Treatment of High Blood Cholesterol in Adults (Adult Treatment Panel III). Third Report of the National Cholesterol Education Program (NCEP) Expert Panel on Detection, Evaluation, and Treatment of High Blood Cholesterol in Adults (Adult Treatment Panel III) Final Report. Circulation 2002;106:3143–421.
4. Wilson PW, D'Agostino RB, Levy D, et al. Prediction of coronary heart disease using risk factor categories. Circulation 1998;97(18):1837–47.
5. Wilson PW. Challenges to improve coronary heart disease risk assessment. JAMA 2009;302(21):2369–70.
6. D'Agostino RB, Grundy SM, Sullivan LM, et al. Validation of the Framingham coronary heart disease prediction scores: results of a multiple ethnic groups investigation. JAMA 2001;286:180–7.
7. Rose G. Sick individuals and sick populations. Int J Epidemiol 1985;14(1):32–8.
8. Greenland P, Knoll MD, Stamler J, et al. Major risk factors as antecedents of fatal and nonfatal coronary heart disease events. JAMA 2003;290(7):891–7.
9. Zethelius B, Berglund L, Sundström J, et al. Use of multiple biomarkers to improve the prediction of death from cardiovascular causes. N Engl J Med 2008;358(20):2107–16.
10. Ridker PM, Buring JE, Rifai N, et al. Development and validation of improved algorithms for the assessment of global cardiovascular risk in women: the reynolds risk score. JAMA 2007;297(6):611–9.

11. Ridker PM, Cook N. Clinical usefulness of very high and very low levels of C-reactive protein across the full range of Framingham risk scores. Circulation 2004; 109(16):1955–9.
12. Ridker PM, Hennekens CH, Buring JE, et al. C-reactive protein and other markers of inflammation in the prediction of cardiovascular disease in women. N Engl J Med 2000;342(12):836–43.
13. Buckley DI, Fu R, Freeman M, et al. C-reactive protein as a risk factor for coronary heart disease: a systematic review and meta-analysis for the U.S. Preventive Services Task Force. Ann Intern Med 2009;151:483–95.
14. Ridker PM, Danielson E, Fonseca FA, et al. Rosuvastatin to prevent vascular events in men and women with elevated c-reactive protein. N Engl J Med 2008;359(21):2195–207.
15. Skalen K, Gustafsson M, Rydberg EK, et al. Subendothelial retention of atherogenic lipoproteins in early atherosclerosis. Nature 2002;417(6890):750–4.
16. Walldius G, Jungner I, Holme I, et al. High apolipoprotein B, low apolipoprotein A-I, and improvement in the prediction of fatal myocardial infarction (AMORIS study): a prospective study. Lancet 2001;358(9298):2026–33.
17. Gotto AM, Whitney E, Stein EA, et al. Relation Between Baseline and On-Treatment Lipid Parameters and First Acute Major Coronary Events in the Air Force/Texas Coronary Atherosclerosis Prevention Study (AFCAPS/TexCAPS). Circulation 2000;101(5):477–84.
18. The Emergency Risk Factors Collaboration, Di Angelantonio E, Sarwar N, et al. Major lipids, apolipoproteins, and risk of vascular disease. JAMA 2009;302(18): 1993–2000.
19. Sniderman AD, Williams K, Contois JH, et al. A meta-analysis of low-density lipoprotein cholesterol, non-high-density lipoprotein cholesterol, and apolipoprotein B as markers of cardiovascular risk. Circ Cardiovasc Qual Outcomes 2011; 4(3):337–45.
20. Ingelsson E, Schaefer EJ, Contois JH, et al. Clinical utility of different lipid measures for prediction of coronary heart disease in men and women. JAMA 2007;298(7):776–85.
21. Kathiresan S, Otvos JD, Sullivan LM, et al. Increased small low-density lipoprotein particle number. Circulation 2006;113(1):20–9.
22. Bennet A, Di Angelantonio E, Erqou S, et al. Lipoprotein(a) levels and risk of future coronary heart disease: large-scale prospective data. Arch Intern Med 2008;168(6):598–608.
23. Bostom A, Cupples L, Jenner J, et al. Elevated plasma lipoprotein(a) and coronary heart disease in men aged 55 year and younger. A prospsective study. JAMA 1996;276(7):544–8.
24. The Emerging Risk Factors Collaboration. Lipoprotein(a) concentration and the risk of coronary heart disease, stroke, and nonvascular mortality. JAMA 2009; 302(4):412–23.
25. Utermann G, Menzel HJ, Kraft HG, et al. Lp(a) glycoprotein phenotypes. Inheritance and relation to Lp(a)-lipoprotein concentrations in plasma. J Clin Invest 1987;80(2):458–65.
26. Omland T, de Lemos JA, Sabatine MS, et al. A sensitive cardiac troponin T assay in stable coronary artery disease. N Engl J Med 2009;361(26):2538–47.
27. Saunders JT, Nambi V, de Lemos JA, et al. Cardiac troponin T measured by a highly sensitive assay predicts coronary heart disease, heart failure, and mortality in the atherosclerosis risk in communities study/clinical perspective. Circulation 2011;123(13):1367–76.

28. deFilippi CR, de Lemos JA, Christenson RH, et al. Association of serial measures of cardiac troponin T using a sensitive assay with incident heart failure and cardiovascular mortality in older adults. JAMA 2010;304(22):2494–502.
29. de Lemos JA, Drazner MH, Omland T, et al. Association of troponin T detected with a highly sensitive assay and cardiac structure and mortality risk in the general population. JAMA 2010;304(22):2503–12.

# LDL Cholesterol:
# The Lower the Better

Seth S. Martin, MD[a], Roger S. Blumenthal, MD[a],
Michael Miller, MD[b],*

KEYWORDS

- Low-density lipoprotein cholesterol • Coronary risk • Statins
- Atherosclerosis

In the face of a high burden of hyperlipidemia and CVD, lipid-lowering therapy has become one of the most important interventions in modern medicine.[1–3] First tested with cholestyramine in the Lipid Research Clinics Coronary Primary Prevention Trial (LRC-CPPT),[4,5] then corroborated with data from statin-based trials,[6] the critical role of LDL-C lowering in CVD risk reduction is firmly established. Decreasing LDL-C has been shown to reduce initial coronary events, recurrent coronary events, and strokes, while slowing progression and even inducing regression of atherosclerosis.

With the tremendous success of LDL-C–lowering therapy, an interesting question has emerged: how low should we go? In this article, the authors tackle this question from multiple complementary perspectives. As such, the article is organized into 3 subsections:

1. Biology, pathophysiology and evolution: lipid biology, the lipid hypothesis, and role of LDL-C in atherosclerosis, and evolutionarily normal cholesterol levels
2. Trials of LDL-C lowering: clinical outcomes studies, plaque-imaging studies
3. Safety data: safety of reducing LDL-C to very low levels with statins.

## BIOLOGY, PATHOPHYSIOLOGY, AND EVOLUTION
### Lipid Biology

Lipoproteins transport cholesterol to peripheral tissue for maintenance of the cell membrane, generation of cellular energy, and metabolism into new bioactive molecules. Cholesterol is a required precursor for bile acid, steroid hormones, and vitamin D. It seems that only very low cholesterol levels are needed to maintain these normal biological

---

The authors have nothing to disclose.

[a] Division of Cardiology, Department of Medicine, Johns Hopkins Ciccarone Center for the Prevention of Heart Disease, 600 North Wolfe Street, Carnegie 565-G, Baltimore, MD 21287, USA

[b] Division of Cardiology, Department of Medicine, Center for Preventive Cardiology, University of Maryland Medical Center, 22 South Greene Street, Room S3B06, Baltimore, MD 21201, USA

* Corresponding author.

E-mail address: mmiller@medicine.umaryland.edu

functions, as patients with heterozygous hypobetalipoproteinemia have LDL-C levels as low as 30 mg/dL without adverse effects.[7] In fact, these patients often exhibit longevity.[7]

Blood cholesterol itself is derived from dietary intake and endogenous hepatic production. Dietary lipids are intestinally absorbed via apolipoprotein B-48 and are then incorporated into chylomicrons. Triglyceride-rich chylomicrons next enter the bloodstream, where they are rapidly hydrolyzed by lipoprotein lipase at the capillary endothelium. Smaller degradation products are principally taken up by the liver, where they are synthesized into the apolipoprotein B-100–containing, triglyceride-rich lipoprotein, very low-density lipoprotein (VLDL). VLDL is broken down by lipoprotein lipase into intermediate-density lipoprotein (IDL). Of note, smaller VLDL particles and IDL may cross the vessel wall to deliver cholesterol to a growing plaque in processes mediated in part by apolipoprotein B-100 and apolipoprotein E.

Further catabolism of VLDL results in cholesterol-rich LDL, the principal determinant of atherosclerosis. The sole protein component of LDL is apolipoprotein B-100, with a single copy per LDL particle. In a pro-oxidative milieu, LDL is oxidized and made recognizable to type A scavenger receptors present on macrophages in the arterial wall. Oxidized LDL plays other critical roles in atherosclerosis, such as increased chemotaxis of inflammatory cells, procoagulation, and reduced responsiveness to nitric oxide–induced vasodilation.[8]

### The lipid hypothesis and role of LDL-C in atherosclerosis

Many patients who die of coronary heart disease (CHD) have elevated blood levels of cholesterol.[9] The Framingham Heart Study, a large population-based cohort study of asymptomatic patients in Massachusetts, first revealed a positive association between total cholesterol and CHD.[10] Subsequently, the Multiple Risk Factor Intervention Trial (MRFIT) showed a J-shaped curvilinear relationship between total cholesterol and CVD mortality.[11] The Johns Hopkins Precursor Study[12] and the Bogulosa Heart Study[13] confirmed that elevated cholesterol in young adulthood is related to CHD later in life. With these observations, combined with animal experiments showing atherosclerosis formation in response to a high-fat diet, early-onset atherosclerosis in genetic variants such as familial hypercholesterolemia, and improved clinical outcomes with lipid lowering, the lipid hypothesis, or LDL hypothesis, emerged as one of the best-supported hypotheses in modern medicine. This hypothesis states that atherosclerosis is causally related to elevated atherogenic cholesterol levels, including LDL-C, and that reduction in blood cholesterol results in decreased incidence of CVD.

From an early age, often by the third decade of life, LDL and other atherogenic lipoprotein particles enter the arterial wall in a gradient-driven process and are retained, and plaque formation begins. Cholesterol, the passenger on the lipoprotein vehicle, is delivered to the intima and inner media of major arteries. Progressively greater amounts of cholesterol are delivered, oxidative and inflammatory responses ensue, and atherosclerosis accumulates. As the natural history of this process ensues over decades, plaque growth eventually becomes so extensive that it can no longer expand in the arterial wall and begins to encroach on the arterial lumen. Therefore, by the time even mild stenosis is visualized on a coronary angiogram, the horse is out of the barn. An acute coronary syndrome (ACS) occurs when the fibrous cap overlying the lipid core ruptures, exposing oxidized lipid and other plaque contents to the bloodstream, resulting in thrombosis and acute disruption of coronary perfusion.

### Evolutionarily normal cholesterol levels

In evolutionary terms, humans are maladapted to handle LDL-C levels in the ranges currently considered normal in modern industrial culture. Consuming high amounts of fatty foods, the mean LDL-C level in the United States population was 115 mg/dL in 2005 to 2006 in The National Health and Nutrition Examination Survey[14] compared with approximately 50 mg/dL in native hunter-gatherers, healthy human neonates, free-living primates, and other wild mammals (**Fig. 1**).[7] Unlike modern Americans, these groups are notably free of CVD. Therefore, it seems CVD is a direct by-product of our societal structure and lifestyles that promote LDL-C levels 2-fold, or more, higher than we were intended to have.

## CLINICAL TRIALS OF LDL-C LOWERING
### Clinical Outcomes Studies

In the mid-1990s results from a series of large clinical outcomes studies became available, which confirmed the efficacy of pharmacologic lipid lowering and reinforced the importance of LDL-C. These randomized trials differed from earlier studies in the use of a new class of pharmacotherapy known as hydroxy-3-methylglutaryl coenzyme A reductase inhibitors, or statins, which inhibit cholesterol biosynthesis, increase hepatic LDL-C uptake, and carry additional beneficial pleiotropic effects.

Initial trials enrolled higher-risk patients for both primary and secondary prevention of CHD. The Scandinavian Simvastatin Survival Study (4S), published in 1994, randomized 4444 CHD patients with total cholesterol between 213 and 309 mg/dL to 20 mg of simvastatin (subsequently titrated) or placebo, and followed the subjects for mortality over a median of 5.4 years.[15] In the simvastatin group, total cholesterol was reduced by 26%, LDL-C was reduced by 36%, and there was a 30% decrease in total mortality (256 vs 182 deaths). In secondary analysis, CHD mortality was reduced by 42%, with similar benefits across quartiles of baseline total cholesterol and LDL-C.[16]

The West of Scotland Coronary Prevention Study (WOSCOPS) extended this finding to the high-risk primary prevention setting.[17] Published in 1995, WOSCOPS randomized 6595 Scottish men without known CHD to 40 mg pravastatin or placebo. Baseline total cholesterol was 272 mg/dL and baseline LDL-C was 192 mg/dL; the study

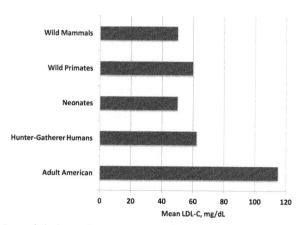

**Fig. 1.** Comparison of cholesterol concentrations from evolutionarily representative groups with those of adult Americans. Mean low-density lipoprotein cholesterol (LDL-C) levels of adult Americans and modern Westernized humans are approximately twice those of evolutionarily normal values. (*Adapted from* O'Keefe JH Jr, Cordain L, Harris WH, et al. Optimal low-density lipoprotein is 50 to 70 mg/dl: lower is better and physiologically normal. J Am Coll Cardiol 2004;43:2143; with permission.)

collected a median of 4.9 years of follow-up data. Pravastatin reduced total cholesterol by 20%, LDL-C by 26%, and CHD events by 31% (248 vs 174 events).

Subsequent trials focused on patients who, during that era of lipidology, were classified as having only mild to moderate elevations in cholesterol. The Cholesterol and Recurrent Events Trial (CARE), published in 1996, randomized 4159 patients with prior heart attacks to 40 mg of pravastatin or placebo and followed them for an average of 5 years.[18] Baseline LDL-C was 139 mg/dL and was reduced by 32% in the pravastatin group. LDL-C levels were maintained at about 97 mg/dL in this group throughout the trial in the pravastatin group, which coincides with a 24% reduction in major coronary events.

In the Long-term Intervention with Pravastatin in Ischaemic Disease (LIPID) trial, published in 1998, 9104 patients with a history of myocardial infarction or unstable angina were randomized to 40 mg pravastatin or placebo, and followed for an average of 6 years.[19] Baseline cholesterol varied from 155 to 271 mg/dL. Reductions in CHD (24%) and all-cause mortality (22%) were associated with a 25% reduction in LDL-C in the pravastatin-allocated group relative to placebo.

The Air Force/Texas Coronary Atherosclerosis Primary Prevention Study (AFCAPS/TexCAPS), published in 1998, reinforced the benefit of statins in primary prevention patients with average levels of cholesterol.[20] The investigators studied 6605 participants who were free of known CVD and had mean LDL-C levels of 150 mg/dL. Participants were randomly assigned to lovastatin (initial dose of 20 mg with subsequent titration) or placebo, and followed for a mean of 5.2 years. Lovastatin-allocated subjects experienced a 25% reduction in LDL-C to 115 mg/dL and a 37% reduction in initial major coronary events (183 vs 113 first events). Despite the consistent success of these early statin trials of the 1990s, more potent statins, lower LDL-C levels, and even better patient outcomes were yet to come.

In 2002 the largest study to date, the Heart Protection Study (HPS), released its findings from 20,536 subjects at increased CVD risk who were randomized to simvastatin and/or antioxidant therapy in a $2 \times 2$ factorial design.[21] After a mean follow-up of 5.5 years, there was a consistent benefit from simvastatin ($\sim$25% proportional event reduction) across a wide array of patient subgroups, including women, patients with diabetes, and patients with baseline LDL-C of less than 100 mg/dL. Simvastatin appeared to provide benefit regardless of baseline LDL-C.

Trials moved on from testing statin versus placebo to evaluating more intensive versus less intensive statin therapy. In the Pravastatin or Atorvastatin Evaluation and Infection Therapy—Thrombolysis in Myocardial Infarction 22 (PROVE IT-TIMI-22) trial,[22] 4162 patients recently hospitalized for an ACS were randomized to atorvastatin, 80 mg or pravastatin, 40 mg to compare intensive with standard lipid-lowering strategies. Mean LDL-C at randomization was 106 mg/dL; on-treatment LDL-C was 95 mg/dL in the pravastatin group and 62 mg/dL in the atorvastatin group. The benefit of high-dose atorvastatin was seen at 30 days and persisted during 2 years of follow-up. There was no identifiable lower LDL-C threshold below which benefit was lost; even the patients attaining LDL-C levels below 40 mg/dL benefited from therapy (**Fig. 2**). This study suggested that optimal on-treatment LDL-C levels are well below those previously achieved, which prompted an extensive footnote to the ATP III guidelines.[2]

In 10,003 patients with stable CHD, the Treating to New Targets (TNT) trial evaluated atorvastatin, 10 mg versus atorvastatin, 80 mg over a mean of 5 years.[23] Baseline LDL-C was 152 mg/dL; on-treatment LDL was 101 mg/dL in the low-dose group and 77 mg/dL in the high-dose group. More intensive atorvastatin yielded a 22% reduction in major coronary events. The Z phase of the Aggrastat to Zocor (A to Z) trial[24] and the

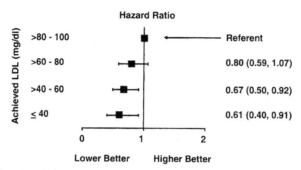

**Fig. 2.** Hazard ratio of the primary end point compared with achieved calculated low-density lipoprotein (LDL) of 80 to 100 mg/dL (adjusted for age, gender, baseline calculated LDL, diabetes mellitus, and prior myocardial infarction). (*From* Wiviott SD, Cannon CP, Morrow DA, et al. Can low-density lipoprotein be too low? The safety and efficacy of achieving very low low-density lipoprotein with intensive statin therapy: a PROVE IT-TIMI 22 substudy. J Am Coll Cardiol 2005;46:1414; with permission.)

Incremental Decrease in End Points through Aggressive Lipid Lowering (IDEAL) trial[25] also tested low-dose versus high-dose strategies in high-risk patients. In A to Z, patients were followed beginning 4 months after suffering an ACS, attained LDL-C levels of 63 mg/dL on high-dose simvastatin, and benefited from a 25% reduction in CVD events. In IDEAL, patients with a history of myocardial infarction lowered LDL-C levels to 79 mg/dL on high-dose statin and experienced a 13% reduction in CVD events.

Most recently, the Justification for the Use of statins in Primary prevention: an Intervention Trial Evaluating Rosuvastatin (JUPITER) trial examined 17,802 participants with normal LDL-C levels (<130 mg/dL; normal for an adult American but not evolutionarily normal) and high-sensitivity C-reactive protein levels of 2 mg/L or greater.[26] Patients were randomized to 20 mg rosuvastatin or placebo, and the rosuvastatin-allocated group attained median LDL-C levels of 55 mg/dL. The trial was stopped early after a median follow-up of 1.9 years because of unequivocal evidence of benefit, including a reduction in the primary end point, each individual CVD end point, and all-cause mortality.

The consistent theme throughout the trials summarized here is that the degree of relative cardiovascular-event reduction is proportional to the degree of LDL-C lowering in both primary (**Fig. 3**) and secondary prevention trials (**Fig. 4**). The Cholesterol Treatment Trialists' 2010 meta-analysis pooled individual participant data from 170,000 randomized subjects in statin trials of more versus less intensive statin regimens and statin versus control.[6] Across a broad range of patient subgroups, statin therapy consistently reduced the annual rate of major cardiovascular events by just over a fifth for each 1.0 mmol/L (39 mg/dL) LDL-C reduction. All-cause mortality was reduced by 10% per 1.0 mmol/L LDL-C reduction (rate ratio [RR], 0.90, 95% confidence interval [CI], 0.87–0.93; $P<.0001$), primarily due to protection from cardiovascular death (RR, 0.80, 99% CI, 0.74–0.87; $P<.0001$). Of importance, there was no evidence of a lower limit of LDL-C below which a reduction did not provide benefit (**Fig. 5**).

## Plaque-Imaging Studies

The Reversing Atherosclerosis with Aggressive Lipid Lowering (REVERSAL) trial examined plaque burden by intravascular ultrasonography at baseline and 18 months

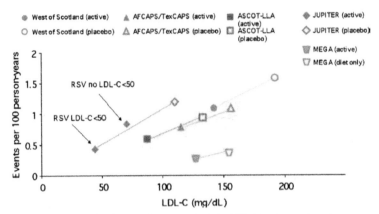

**Fig. 3.** Relation of major cardiovascular event rate to LDL-C at 1 year in primary prevention trials. Placebo groups are indicated by open symbols, and statin groups by solid symbols. Clinical events: West of Scotland (blue circles) and ASCOT-LLA (green squares), myocardial infarction (MI)/coronary heart disease (CHD) death; AFCAPS/TexCAPs (orange triangles), fatal and nonfatal MI, unstable angina, sudden death; MEGA (blue baskets), fatal and nonfatal MI, angina, cardiac and sudden death, revascularization; JUPITER (purple diamonds), MI, stroke, cardiovascular death, arterial revascularization, unstable angina. Rosuvastatin (RSV)-treated participants without low-density lipoprotein cholesterol (LDL-C) less than 50 mg/dL (median 69 mg/dL) and with LDL-C less than 50 mg/dL (median 44 mg/dL) are plotted separately. AFCAPS/TexCAPS, Air Force/Texas Coronary Atherosclerosis Prevention Study; ASCOT-LLA, Anglo-Scandinavian Cardiac Outcomes Trial—Lipid-Lowering Arm; JUPITER, Justification for the Use of Statins in Prevention: an Intervention Trial Evaluating Rosuvastatin; MEGA, Management of Elevated Cholesterol in the Primary Prevention Group of Adult Japanese. (*From* Hsia J, MacFadyen JG, Monyak J, et al. Cardiovascular event reduction and adverse events among subjects attaining low-density lipoprotein cholesterol <50 mg/dl with rosuvastatin. The JUPITER trial (Justification for the Use of Statins in Prevention: an Intervention Trial Evaluating Rosuvastatin). J Am Coll Cardiol 2011;57:1673; with permission.)

in a low-dose versus high-dose statin study design.[27] A total of 502 patients with symptomatic CHD were randomized to simvastatin, 40 mg versus atorvastatin, 80 mg, and results were published in 2004. High-dose atorvastatin resulted in greater lowering of LDL-C (79 mg/dL vs 110 mg/dL) and was associated with halted atherosclerosis, whereas patients receiving 40 mg simvastatin experienced progression in plaque. Combined with other early studies, data suggested that atherosclerosis does not progress when LDL is 67 mg/dL or less (**Fig. 6**).

In A Study to Evaluate the Effect of Rosuvastatin on Intravascular Ultrasound-Derived Coronary Atheroma Burden (ASTEROID), published in 2006, 507 patients with angiographic CHD were treated with 40 mg rosuvastatin.[28] LDL-C was reduced from baseline 130 mg/dL to 61 mg/dL over 2 years, with 75% of patients achieving LDL-C less than 70 mg/dL. At the conclusion of the study, 64% of patients achieved atherosclerosis regression.

The Measuring Effects on Intima-Media Thickness: An Evaluation of Rosuvastatin (METEOR) trial extended these results into the primary prevention setting.[29] In METEOR, 984 asymptomatic low-risk patients were randomized to 40 mg rosuvastatin or placebo. Patients receiving rosuvastatin attained LDL-C levels of 78 mg/dL, compared with 152 mg/dL in the placebo group. Statin-allocated subjects demonstrated net atherosclerosis regression versus progression in the placebo group.

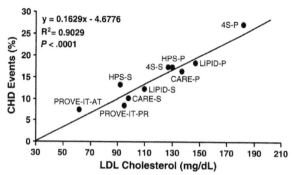

**Fig. 4.** Coronary heart disease (CHD) event rates in secondary prevention trials (5 years in duration except the PROVE-IT study, which lasted 2 years) were directly proportional to low-density lipoprotein (LDL) cholesterol levels. The event rate is predicted to approach 0 at LDL of 30 mg/dL. 4S, Scandinavian Simvastatin Survival Study; CARE, Cholesterol And Recurrent Events trial; HPS, Heart Protection Study; LIPID, Long-term Intervention with Pravastatin In Ischemic Disease trial; PROVE-IT, PRavastatin Or atorVastatin Evaluation and Infection Therapy trial. Other abbreviations are as in **Fig. 6**. (*From* O'Keefe JH Jr, Cordain L, Harris WH, et al. Optimal low-density lipoprotein is 50 to 70 mg/dl: lower is better and physiologically normal. J Am Coll Cardiol 2004;43:2144; with permission.)

In the Study of Coronary Atheroma by Intravascular Ultrasound: Effect of Rosuvastatin versus Atorvastatin (SATURN), investigators performed serial intravascular ultrasonography at baseline and after 104 weeks of treatment in 1039 CHD patients randomly assigned to treatment with atorvastatin, 80 mg daily or rosuvastatin, 40 mg daily.[30] On average, the rosuvastatin group attained LDL-C levels of 63 mg/dL and the atorvastatin group attained levels of 70 mg/dL. Coronary atherosclerosis, as quantified by percent atheroma volume, regressed with each treatment strategy: by 0.99% (95% CI, −1.19 to −0.63) with atorvastatin and by 1.2% (95% CI, −1.52 to −0.90) with rosuvastatin. Both agents induced regression in most patients: 63% with atorvastatin and 68.5% with rosuvastatin.

## Residual Risk and Combination Lipid-Lowering Therapy

After first emphasizing appropriately potent statin therapy based on the aforementioned extensive data, and lifestyle changes, additional lipid-lowering agents (eg, bile acid sequestrants, niacin, and ezetimibe) can be considered to assist patients in achieving lower LDL-C levels. Although this is a logical strategy, favorable outcomes data for nonstatin lipid-lowering agents generally preceded the statin era, with more recent studies focused on surrogate end points, and thus their efficacy as add-on therapy is yet to be demonstrated in large, randomized clinical outcomes trials. Nevertheless, despite risk reduction with aggressive statin therapy, some patients do not achieve their LDL-C goal, and certain groups of patients, such as those with metabolic syndrome, diabetes mellitus, high non–high-density lipoprotein cholesterol (HDL-C), and low HDL-C, have a particularly high residual risk on statin therapy.[31] Therefore, in addition to global risk-reduction strategies, there is great interest in nonstatin lipid-lowering agents and HDL-raising therapies, although the latter are beyond the scope of this article.

Bile acid sequestrants favorably redirect enterohepatic exchange of bile acids, which is associated with increased expression of hepatic LDL-C receptors and clearance of circulating LDL-C, leading to a 5% to 30% dose-dependent reduction in

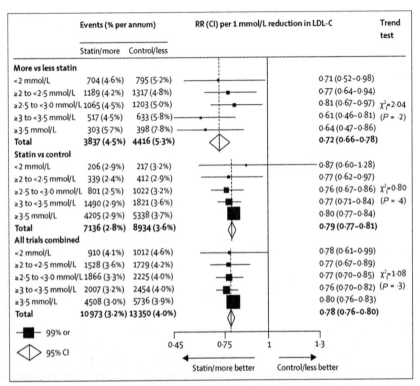

**Fig. 5.** Effects on major vascular events per 1.0 mmol/L (39 mg/dL) reduction in LDL cholesterol (LDL-C), by baseline LDL-C concentration on the less intensive or control regimen. Rate ratios (RRs) are plotted for each comparison of first-event rates between treatment groups, and are weighted per 1.0 mmol/L (39 mg/dL) LDL-C difference at 1 year. Analyses were done with trial-specific and subgroup-specific LDL weights for each baseline LDL-C category. Missing data are not plotted. RRs are shown, with horizontal lines denoting 99% confidence intervals (CIs) or with open diamonds showing 95% CIs. (*From* Cholesterol Treatment Trialists' (CTT) Collaboration, Baigent C, Blackwell L, Emberson J, et al. Efficacy and safety of more intensive lowering of LDL cholesterol: a meta-analysis of data from 170,000 participants in 26 randomised trials. Lancet 2010;376:1676; with permission.)

LDL-C concentration. These drugs have no systemic absorption; remaining in the gut, they may be associated with gastrointestinal disturbances (eg, constipation) and can impair absorption of other drugs. The LRC-CPPT trial[4,5] showed significant reductions in myocardial infarction and cardiovascular death with bile acid sequestrant monotherapy; however, combination therapy trials are lacking.

Niacin is touted most for raising HDL-C levels, but it also reduces hepatic VLDL cholesterol output, thereby reducing atherogenic LDL-C in a dose-dependent manner. In the Coronary Drug Project, niacin monotherapy provided protection from myocardial infarction and reduced long-term mortality by 11% at 15 years.[32] Although niacin did not show a benefit in patients with low LDL-C (~71 mg/dL) on statins ± ezetimibe in The Atherothrombosis Intervention in Metabolic Syndrome with Low HDL/High Triglycerides: Impact on Global Health Outcomes (AIM-HIGH) study,[33] the much larger Treatment of HDL to Reduce the Incidence of Vascular Events (HPS-2-THRIVE) trial is ongoing, with results expected in 2013.

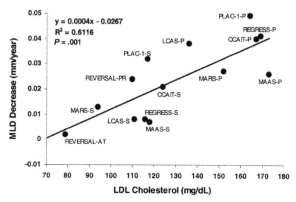

**Fig. 6.** Atherosclerosis progression varies directly with low-density lipoprotein (LDL) cholesterol. This regression line indicates that atherosclerosis does not progress when LDL is 67 mg/dL or less. Data from randomized placebo-controlled trials using statins for preventing atherosclerosis progression were used for computation of the univariate regression lines correlating LDL with outcomes. Regression estimates, model $R^2$, and $P$ values for LDL effect were obtained from the unweighted regression lines. AT, atorvastatin; CCAIT, Canadian Coronary Atherosclerosis Intervention Trial; LCAS, Lipoprotein and Coronary Atherosclerosis Study; MAAS, Multicentre Anti-Atheroma Study; MARS, Monitored Atherosclerosis Regression Study; MLD, mean luminal diameter; P, placebo; PLAC, Pravastatin Limitation of Atherosclerosis in the Coronary Arteries study; PR, pravastatin; REGRESS, Regression Growth Evaluation Statin Study; REVERSAL, Reversal of Atherosclerosis with Aggressive Lipid Lowering; S, statin. (*From* O'Keefe JH Jr, Cordain L, Harris WH, et al. Optimal low-density lipoprotein is 50 to 70 mg/dl: lower is better and physiologically normal. J Am Coll Cardiol 2004;43:2144; with permission.)

Ezetimibe reduces LDL-C by 15% to 20% primarily by impeding cholesterol absorption at the brush border of the intestine. The ezetimibe-statin combination enhances achievement of target LDL-C goals.[34] However, surrogate end-point trials, possibly limited by the end point itself, have introduced uncertainty and confusion. In the Ezetimibe and Simvastatin in Hypercholesterolemia Enhances Atherosclerosis Regression (ENHANCE) trial,[35] involving 720 patients with heterozygous familial hypercholesterolemia, the addition of ezetimibe to maximal simvastatin therapy yielded greater LDL-C reduction (56% vs 39%), but there was no difference in carotid intima-media thickness at 2 years. Reporting a discordant result, the Arterial Biology for the Investigation of the Treatment Effects of Reducing Cholesterol 6—HDL and LDL Treatment Strategies (ARBITER 6-HALTS) study observed a paradoxic increase in carotid intima-media thickness with LDL-C lowering by ezetimibe.[36] The Study of Heart and Renal Protection (SHARP) trial[37] provided the first look at an ezetimibe trial powered for clinical outcomes and found that the drug added to simvastatin reduced CVD events, although the comparator group was allocated placebo, not statin monotherapy. Improved Reduction of Outcomes: Vytorin Efficacy International Trial (IMPROVE-IT), a large clinical trial adding ezetimibe to simvastatin monotherapy in approximately 18,000 patients following ACSs, anticipates completion in 2013.

## SAFETY DATA ON REDUCING LDL-C TO VERY LOW LEVELS WITH STATINS

Intervening pharmacologically to reduce LDL-C to what are considered very low levels by modern standards, but are generally within the evolutionarily physiologic range (see earlier discussion), seems to be a safe strategy based on data from thousands of patients studied during the last several decades. Most of these data are derived from treatment with statin, a class of drugs with an excellent safety profile at standard doses and with side effects that are rarely irreversible. With this backdrop, and the status of statins as first-line therapy, this section focuses on the safety of reducing LDL-C to very low levels with statins.

Myopathy is commonly considered in clinical practice. A systematic overview of risks associated with statin therapy from 35 randomized clinical trials including 74,102 participants with a mean follow-up of 17 months (range 1.5–64.8 months) found no significant increase in the risk of myalgias, creatine kinase elevations, rhabdomyolysis, or discontinuation of statin therapy because of any adverse event.[38] Safety data from randomized controlled trials is biased by the fact that many of these trials had run-in phases that selected patients who are prone to early adverse effects from statin therapy. Nevertheless, in patients who tolerate statin therapy well during the initiation period, the aforementioned data indicate that statin therapy is extremely safe.

In routine clinical practice, 8% to 9% of statin-treated versus 4% to 6% of untreated patients experience myopathic events, of which 95% are myalgias or mild myositis.[39] Rhabdomyolysis is a rare, severe form of myopathy, with myoglobin release into the circulation and risk of renal failure, occurring in fewer than 1 per 10,000 patients on statin therapy.[40] It seems to mostly occur in the setting of drug-drug interactions and certain comorbidities (**Table 1**). In fact, side effects of statin, including muscle toxicity, are not significantly related to on-treatment LDL-C level (**Table 2**).[7] When they occur, statin discontinuation generally leads to full recovery.

A systematic review of 74,102 participants did identify an increased risk of transaminase elevations with statin therapy.[38] Asymptomatic transaminitis appears to be a statin-based class effect, but is not strongly tied to an increased risk of liver disease.[40] Alanine transaminase elevations exceeding 3 times the upper limit of normal have occurred in 0.11% to 3.3% of patients on statin therapy.[40] In patients with mild to moderately abnormal liver tests at baseline, statin therapy is safe and can improve liver tests, potentially attributable to nonalcoholic fatty liver disease.[41]

Statins may also be linked to a modest increase in the incidence of type 2 diabetes mellitus (T2DM). For example, a 9% increase (odds ratio, 1.09; 95% CI, 1.02–1.17) in

**Table 1**
**Major safety and efficacy outcomes across strata of achieved LDL-C (percentage of subjects)**

| Concomitant Medications | Other Conditions |
| --- | --- |
| Fibrate | Advanced age (especially >80 y) |
| Nicotinic acid (rarely) | Women > men especially at older age |
| Cyclosporine | Small body frame, frailty |
| Antifungal azoles | Multisystem disease |
| Macrolide antibiotics | Multiple medications |
| HIV protease inhibitors | Perioperative period |
| Nefazadone | Alcohol abuse |
| Verapamil, Amiodarone | Grapefruit juice (>1 L/d) |

*Abbreviation:* HIV, human immunodeficiency virus.
*From* Wiviott SD, Cannon CP, Morrow DA, et al. Can low-density lipoprotein be too low? The safety and efficacy of achieving very low low-density lipoprotein with intensive statin therapy: a PROVE IT-TIMI 22 substudy. J Am Coll Cardiol 2005;46:1414; with permission.

**Table 2**
**Risk factors for the development of myopathy**

| Safety Measure | Achieved LDL-C (mg/dL) | | | | P Trend |
|---|---|---|---|---|---|
| | >80–100 n = 256 | >60–80 n = 576 | >40–60 n = 631 | <40 n = 193 | |
| Muscle Side Effects[a] | | | | | |
| Myalgia | 6.4 | 4.3 | 6.2 | 5.7 | .75 |
| Myositis | 0.4 | 0.6 | 0.6 | 0 | .64 |
| CK >3× ULN | 2.3 | 0.7 | 1.9 | 1.0 | .18 |
| CK >10× ULN | 0 | 0 | 0.3 | 0 | .45 |
| Rhabdomyolysis | 0 | 0 | 0 | 0 | 1.0 |
| Liver Side Effects | | | | | |
| ALT >3× ULN | 3.2 | 3.0 | 3.2 | 2.6 | .98 |
| Study drug discontinued because of LFT | 2.0 | 2.6 | 2.4 | 1.6 | .83 |
| Other | | | | | |
| Hemorrhagic stroke | 0.4 | 0.2 | 0 | 0 | .12 |
| Retinal AE | 0.4 | 0.9 | 1.0 | 0 | .48 |
| Suicide/trauma death | 0 | 0 | 0 | 0 | 1.0 |
| Study drug discontinued because of any AE | 10.2 | 9.4 | 9.7 | 9.8 | .99 |
| Major Efficacy Measures | | | | | |
| Death | 1.1 | 1.4 | 1.3 | 0.5 | .59 |
| CHD death | 0.5 | 0.5 | 0.6 | 0.0 | .06 |
| Myocardial infarction | 1.0 | 0.7 | 0.5 | 0.6 | .009 |
| Any stroke | 0.8 | 0.9 | 0.6 | 1.6 | .32 |
| Primary composite[a] | 26.1 | 22.2 | 20.4 | 20.4 | .10 |

*Abbreviations:* AE, adverse event; ALT, alanine aminotransferase; CHD, coronary heart disease; CK, creatine kinase; LFT, liver function test; LDL-C, low-density lipoprotein cholesterol; ULN, upper limit of normal.

[a] Primary composite: percent of subjects with any of the following: death, myocardial infarction, stroke, unstable angina requiring rehospitalization, and revascularization. Myalgia: muscle symptoms without CK elevation. Myositis: muscle symptoms with CK elevation. Rhabdomyolysis: muscle symptoms with CK >10 × ULN and evidence of renal dysfunction.

*Adapted from* Pasternak RC, Smith SC Jr, Bairey-Merz CN, et al. ACC/AHA/NHLBI clinical advisory on the use and safety of statins. Circulation 2002;106:1027; with permission.

incident T2DM was reported in a meta-analysis of 13 trials encompassing 91,140 participants[42] with an approximate new case of diabetes per 1000 person-years of treatment. Although the precise mechanism has yet to be elucidated, the overall risk of statin-mediated T2DM is low in absolute terms and relative to the reduction in CVD events.

Despite some concerns, there is little evidentiary data demonstrating an increase in malignancy rates or memory loss associated with statin use. By contrast, advanced chronic illnesses, including carcinoma, are associated with very low LDL-C levels, especially in the setting of malnutrition. Previously this association raised safety concerns that aggressive LDL-C lowering might enhance the risk of malignancy, but this fear has not been borne out in subsequent analyses.[6,43] Likewise, there is evidence pointing against a causative relation between statins and cognitive decline.[44]

Overall, the potential harm of statin therapy does not overshadow established benefits in the vast majority of statin-treated patients. Transaminases can be routinely monitored and creatine kinase levels can be checked in the setting of muscle complaints. Practitioners should pay attention to potential drug-drug interactions and conditions that put patients at higher risk for these side effects. The Food and Drug Administration continues to actively collect data on adverse effects of statins and other lipid-lowering agents through the Adverse Events Reporting System. In JUPITER, those participants attaining LDL-C levels of less than 50 mg/dL experienced a reduction in CVD events and all-cause mortality without a systematic increase in reported adverse events.[45] Framing the benefits of aggressive LDL-C lowering with statin therapy against their competing risk, the National Lipid Association Statin Safety Task Force stated: "For every 1 million high-risk persons treated with a statin over 100,000 heart attacks, strokes or other major adverse cardiac event will be prevented for every 1 serious side effect. Therefore, the person should fear the heart attack not the statin."[46]

## SUMMARY

LDL-C has a primary role in the pathogenesis and epidemiology of CVD. Optimal LDL-C levels are less than 70 mg/dL, if not lower, based on pathobiology, evolution, and extensive data from clinical trials. Such levels are associated with protection from CVD and atherosclerosis regression without major safety concerns. At present, a threshold has not been found below which patients do not benefit from lowering of LDL-C. Therefore, when managing patients' LDL-C levels, the prevailing dogma is the lower the LDL-C, the better!

## REFERENCES

1. Executive summary of the third report of the National Cholesterol Education Program (NCEP) expert panel on detection, evaluation, and treatment of high blood cholesterol in adults (Adult Treatment Panel III). JAMA 2001;285:2486–97.
2. Grundy SM, Cleeman JI, Merz CN, et al. Implications of recent clinical trials for the National Cholesterol Education Program Adult Treatment Panel III guidelines. Circulation 2004;110:227–39.
3. Lloyd-Jones D, Adams R, Carnethon M, et al. Heart disease and stroke statistics—2009 update: a report from the American Heart Association Statistics Committee and Stroke Statistics Subcommittee. Circulation 2009;119:480–6.
4. The Lipid Research Clinics Coronary Primary Prevention Trial results. I. Reduction in incidence of coronary heart disease. JAMA 1984;251:351–64.
5. The Lipid Research Clinics Coronary Primary Prevention Trial results. II. The relationship of reduction in incidence of coronary heart disease to cholesterol lowering. JAMA 1984;251:365–74.
6. Baigent C, Blackwell L, Emberson J, et al. Efficacy and safety of more intensive lowering of LDL cholesterol: a meta-analysis of data from 170,000 participants in 26 randomised trials. Lancet 2010;376:1670–81.
7. O'Keefe JH Jr, Cordain L, Harris WH, et al. Optimal low-density lipoprotein is 50 to 70 mg/dL: lower is better and physiologically normal. J Am Coll Cardiol 2004;43:2142–6.
8. Witztum JL, Steinberg D. Role of oxidized low density lipoprotein in atherogenesis. J Clin Invest 1991;88:1785–92.
9. Greenland P, Knoll MD, Stamler J, et al. Major risk factors as antecedents of fatal and nonfatal coronary heart disease events. JAMA 2003;290:891–7.

10. Kannel WB, Castelli WP, Gordon T, et al. Serum cholesterol, lipoproteins, and the risk of coronary heart disease. The Framingham study. Ann Intern Med 1971;74: 1–12.
11. Neaton JD, Wentworth D. Serum cholesterol, blood pressure, cigarette smoking, and death from coronary heart disease. Overall findings and differences by age for 316,099 white men. Multiple Risk Factor Intervention Trial Research Group. Arch Intern Med 1992;152:56–64.
12. Pearson TA, LaCroix AZ, Mead LA, et al. The prediction of midlife coronary heart disease and hypertension in young adults: the Johns Hopkins multiple risk equations. Am J Prev Med 1990;6:23–8.
13. Berenson GS, Srinivasan SR, Bao W, et al. Association between multiple cardiovascular risk factors and atherosclerosis in children and young adults. The Bogalusa Heart Study. N Engl J Med 1998;338:1650–6.
14. Kuklina EV, Yoon PW, Keenan NL. Trends in high levels of low-density lipoprotein cholesterol in the United States, 1999-2006. JAMA 2009;302:2104–10.
15. Randomised trial of cholesterol lowering in 4444 patients with coronary heart disease: the Scandinavian Simvastatin Survival Study (4S). Lancet 1994;344:1383–9.
16. Baseline serum cholesterol and treatment effect in the Scandinavian Simvastatin Survival Study (4S). Lancet 1995;345:1274–5.
17. Shepherd J, Cobbe SM, Ford I, et al. Prevention of coronary heart disease with pravastatin in men with hypercholesterolemia. West of Scotland Coronary Prevention Study Group. N Engl J Med 1995;333:1301–7.
18. Sacks FM, Pfeffer MA, Moye LA, et al. The effect of pravastatin on coronary events after myocardial infarction in patients with average cholesterol levels. Cholesterol and Recurrent Events Trial investigators. N Engl J Med 1996;335: 1001–9.
19. Prevention of cardiovascular events and death with pravastatin in patients with coronary heart disease and a broad range of initial cholesterol levels. The Long-Term Intervention with Pravastatin in Ischaemic Disease (LIPID) Study Group. N Engl J Med 1998;339:1349–57.
20. Downs JR, Clearfield M, Weis S, et al. Primary prevention of acute coronary events with lovastatin in men and women with average cholesterol levels: results of AFCAPS/TexCAPS. Air Force/Texas Coronary Atherosclerosis Prevention Study. JAMA 1998;279:1615–22.
21. MRC/BHF Heart Protection Study of cholesterol lowering with simvastatin in 20,536 high-risk individuals: a randomised placebo-controlled trial. Lancet 2002;360:7–22.
22. Cannon CP, Braunwald E, McCabe CH, et al. Intensive versus moderate lipid lowering with statins after acute coronary syndromes. N Engl J Med 2004;350: 1495–504.
23. LaRosa JC, Grundy SM, Waters DD, et al. Intensive lipid lowering with atorvastatin in patients with stable coronary disease. N Engl J Med 2005;352:1425–35.
24. de Lemos JA, Blazing MA, Wiviott SD, et al. Early intensive vs a delayed conservative simvastatin strategy in patients with acute coronary syndromes: phase Z of the A to Z trial. JAMA 2004;292:1307–16.
25. Pedersen TR, Faergeman O, Kastelein JJ, et al. High-dose atorvastatin vs usual-dose simvastatin for secondary prevention after myocardial infarction: the IDEAL study: a randomized controlled trial. JAMA 2005;294:2437–45.
26. Ridker PM, Danielson E, Fonseca FA, et al. Rosuvastatin to prevent vascular events in men and women with elevated C-reactive protein. N Engl J Med 2008;359:2195–207.

27. Nissen SE, Tuzcu EM, Schoenhagen P, et al. Effect of intensive compared with moderate lipid-lowering therapy on progression of coronary atherosclerosis: a randomized controlled trial. JAMA 2004;291:1071–80.

28. Nissen SE, Nicholls SJ, Sipahi I, et al. Effect of very high-intensity statin therapy on regression of coronary atherosclerosis: the ASTEROID trial. JAMA 2006;295:1556–65.

29. Crouse JR 3rd, Raichlen JS, Riley WA, et al. Effect of rosuvastatin on progression of carotid intima-media thickness in low-risk individuals with subclinical athero-sclerosis: the METEOR Trial. JAMA 2007;297:1344–53.

30. Nicholls SJ, Ballantyne CM, Barter PJ, et al. Effect of two intensive statin regimens on progression of coronary disease. N Engl J Med 2011;365:2078–87.

31. Campbell CY, Rivera JJ, Blumenthal RS. Residual risk in statin-treated patients: future therapeutic options. Curr Cardiol Rep 2007;9:499–505.

32. Canner PL, Berge KG, Wenger NK, et al. Fifteen year mortality in coronary drug project patients: long-term benefit with niacin. J Am Coll Cardiol 1986;8:1245–55.

33. Boden WE, Probstfield JL, Anderson T, et al. Niacin in patients with low HDL choles-terol levels receiving intensive statin therapy. N Engl J Med 2011;365:2255–67.

34. Mikhailidis DP, Lawson RW, McCormick AL, et al. Comparative efficacy of the addi-tion of ezetimibe to statin vs statin titration in patients with hypercholesterolaemia: systematic review and meta-analysis. Curr Med Res Opin 2011;27:1191–210.

35. Kastelein JJ, Akdim F, Stroes ES, et al. Simvastatin with or without ezetimibe in familial hypercholesterolemia. N Engl J Med 2008;358:1431–43.

36. Taylor AJ, Villines TC, Stanek EJ, et al. Extended-release niacin or ezetimibe and carotid intima-media thickness. N Engl J Med 2009;361:2113–22.

37. Baigent C, Landray MJ, Reith C, et al. The effects of lowering LDL cholesterol with simvastatin plus ezetimibe in patients with chronic kidney disease (Study of Heart and Renal Protection): a randomised placebo-controlled trial. Lancet 2011;377: 2181–92.

38. Kashani A, Phillips CO, Foody JM, et al. Risks associated with statin therapy: a systematic overview of randomized clinical trials. Circulation 2006;114:2788–97.

39. Nichols GA, Koro CE. Does statin therapy initiation increase the risk for myop-athy? an observational study of 32,225 diabetic and nondiabetic patients. Clin Ther 2007;29:1761–70.

40. Armitage J. The safety of statins in clinical practice. Lancet 2007;370:1781–90.

41. Athyros VG, Tziomalos K, Gossios TD, et al. Safety and efficacy of long-term statin treatment for cardiovascular events in patients with coronary heart disease and abnormal liver tests in the Greek Atorvastatin and Coronary Heart Disease Evaluation (GREACE) Study: a post-hoc analysis. Lancet 2010;376:1916–22.

42. Sattar N, Preiss D, Murray HM, et al. Statins and risk of incident diabetes: a collab-orative meta-analysis of randomised statin trials. Lancet 2010;375:735–42.

43. Dale KM, Coleman CI, Henyan NN, et al. Statins and cancer risk: a meta-analysis. JAMA 2006;295:74–80.

44. Muldoon MF, Barger SD, Ryan CM, et al. Effects of lovastatin on cognitive function and psychological well-being. Am J Med 2000;108:538–46.

45. Hsia J, MacFadyen JG, Monyak J, et al. Cardiovascular event reduction and adverse events among subjects attaining low-density lipoprotein cholesterol <50 mg/dl with rosuvastatin. The JUPITER trial (Justification for the Use of Statins in Prevention: an Intervention Trial Evaluating Rosuvastatin). J Am Coll Cardiol 2011;57:1666–75.

46. McKenney JM, Davidson MH, Jacobson TA, et al. Final conclusions and recom-mendations of the National Lipid Association Statin Safety Assessment Task Force. Am J Cardiol 2006;97:89C–94C.

# HDL–Cholesterol: Perfection is the Enemy of Good?

Ragavendra R. Baliga, MD, MBA

---

**KEYWORDS**

- High-density lipoprotein • Cholesterol • Cardiovascular disease
- Atherosclerosis

---

Intensive low-density lipoprotein (LDL) lowering with statins (even in the presence of significant atherosclerosis) reduces the risk of major atherosclerotic cardiovascular events by approximately 40% to 50%.[1–6] This means that 50% to 60% of risk remains, and this is referred to as residual risk. Strategies to reduce this residual risk include increasing high-density lipoprotein–cholesterol (HDL-C) levels because increased HDL-C is associated with favorable outcomes in atherosclerotic cardiovascular disease[7,8] and HDL-C is reported to be the strongest predictor of coronary heart disease (CHD) risk reduction in a review of 17 prospective, randomized lipid trials of more than 44,000 patients, presented at the American Heart Association Annual Meeting 2004.[9] Every change of 10 mg/dL in the HDL-C level is associated with a 50% change in risk (based on the elderly cohort of the Framingham Heart Study).[10] For every 1 mg/dL increase in HDL-C, there is a 2% decrease in risk of CHD in men and a 3% decrease in women, according to one meta-analysis.[11] There is a strong inverse relationship between HDL levels and cardiovascular risk. Given the importance of HDL-C levels, The New Zealand Guidelines group has incorporated HDL in its cardiovascular risk assessment (**Fig. 1**).

The Framingham Heart Study showed that, as HDL-C decreases, it contributes significantly to CHD risk at all levels of LDL-C (**Fig. 2**).[12] HDL-C is also a predictor of cardiovascular events at 5 years even when LDL-C is less than 70 mg/dL. An analysis of PROSPER (Prospective Study of Pravastatin in the Elderly at Risk) study data indicated further that a specific subgroup received most of the benefit; that is, those with an HDL-C of less than 1.15 mmol/L (<45 mg/dL) or an LDL-C/HDL-C ratio greater than 3.3.[13] In such individuals, the risk reduction for coronary events was 33% rather than the 19% seen in the whole cohort. Focusing on this subgroup reduces the number needed to treat (NNT) to prevent 1 coronary event from 40 to 17. However, efforts to increase HDL-C with pharmacotherapy have not yet been shown to be associated with better outcomes, particularly in patients in whom significant risk reduction has already been achieved by lowering LDL levels with statin therapy.[1,2,14] The quest for HDL-increasing agents that have incremental, improved, cardiovascular outcomes

---

Division of Cardiovascular Medicine, The Ohio State University, Columbus, OH 43054, USA
*E-mail address:* rrbaliga@gmail.com

Med Clin N Am 96 (2012) 27–37
doi:10.1016/j.mcna.2012.01.001
0025-7125/12/$ – see front matter © 2012 Published by Elsevier Inc.

**A**

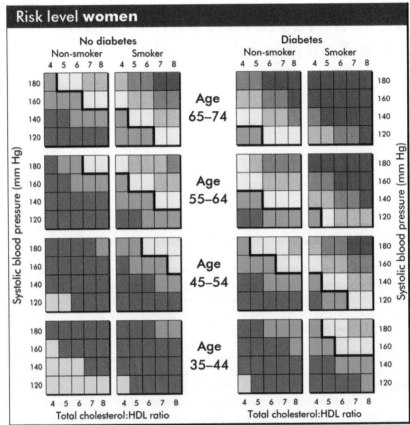

## Risk level **women**

Risk level (for women and men)
5-year cardiovascular disease (CVD) risk (fatal and non-fatal)

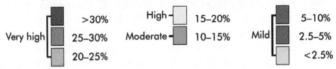

Very high: >30%, 25–30%, 20–25%
High: 15–20%, Moderate: 10–15%
Mild: 5–10%, 2.5–5%, <2.5%

**How to use the Charts**

- Identify the chart relating to the person's sex, diabetic status, smoking history and age.
- Within the chart choose the cell nearest to the person's age, systolic blood pressure (SBP) and total cholesterol (TC) TC:HDL ratio. For example, the lower left cell contains all non-smokers without diabetes who are 35–44 years and have a TC:HDL ratio of less than 4.5 and a SBP of less than 130 mm Hg. People who fall exactly on a threshold between cells are placed in the cell indicating higher risk.
- The risk charts now include values for SBP alone, as this is the most informative of conventionally measured blood pressure parameters for cardiovascular risk. Diastolic pressures may add some predictive power, especially at younger ages (eg, a diastolic pressure consistently >100 mm Hg in a patient with SBP values between 140 and 170 mm Hg).

**Fig. 1.** Risk assessment tool devised by a New Zealand task force to determine 5-year total cardiovascular disease (CVD) risk based on age, sex, smoking history, lipid and glucose levels, and blood pressure: (*A*) for women; (*B*) for men. HDL, high-density lipoprotein; TC, total cholesterol. (*From* New Zealand Guidelines Group. New Zealand Cardiovascular Guidelines Handbook: A summary resource for primary care practitioners. 2nd ed. Wellington: New Zealand Guidelines Group; 2009. Available at: http://www.nzgg.org.nz/library_resources/45_new_zealand_cardiovascular_guidelines_handbook:_a_summary_resource_for_primary_care_practitioners. © 2009 Ministry of Health; used with permission.)

**B**

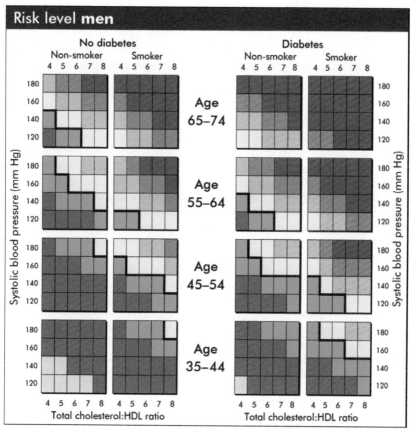

**Fig. 1.** (*continued*)

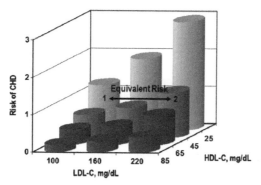

**Fig. 2.** Low HDL-C is associated with increased CHD risk at all levels of LDL-C: The Framingham Study. Although patient 1 has lower LDL-C (100 mg/dL) with HDL-C 25 mg/dL, and patient 2 has a much higher LDL-C of 220 mg/dL, with HDL-C 45 mg/dL, they both have an equivalent risk of coronary heart disease because higher HDL-C is associated with lower risk. (*Data from* Castelli WP. Cholesterol and lipids in the risk of coronary artery disease–the Framingham Heart Study. Can J Cardiol 1988;4(Suppl A):5A–10A.)

is currently ongoing and this is supported by post hoc analysis that suggests that HDL-C levels predict cardiovascular events in patients on statin therapy even when LDL-C levels are less than 70 mg/dL.[15] In the third National Health and Nutrition Examination Survey (NHANES III), low HDL-C was reported in 35% of men (<40 mg/dL) and 39% of women (<50 mg/dL).[16] Therefore, the inverse relationship between HDL-C levels and atherosclerotic cardiovascular disease makes strategies to increase HDL a worthwhile investigative effort.

## WHAT IS HDL?

HDLs are the densest and smallest of the plasma lipoproteins. HDL particles are either spherical or discoidal.[17] Most of the particles are spherical and consist of a fatty core (mainly cholesteryl esters with a small amount of triglyceride) surrounded by an outer layer of phospholipids, free (nonesterified) cholesterol, and apolipoproteins. Discoidal HDL particles are in the minority and are composed of surface constituents arranged as a molecular bilayer consisting of phospholipids and free cholesterol encircled by apolipoproteins. These discoidal particles are a nascent form of HDLs that usually exist only for a limited period in the circulation before being rapidly converted into the spherical form.

## CLASSIFICATION OF HDLs

HDLs are classified based on size, charge, apolipoprotein composition, and separation by hydrated density. Density gradient ultracentrifugation separates HDL into large spherical $HDL_2$, small, dense, spherical $HDL_3$, and very high-density lipoprotein. Gradient gel electrophoresis separates HDL into $HDL_{2a}$, $HDL_{2b}$, $HDL_{3a}$, $HDL_{3b}$, and $HDL_{3c}$. Two-dimensional gel electrophoresis separates HDL particles into the lipid-poor pre-$\beta_1$, pre-$\beta_2$, mature cholesteryl ester–containing $\alpha$-HDL ($\alpha_1$–$\alpha_4$), and pre-$\beta_2$ lipoproteins (see **Fig. 2**). Based on apolipoprotein composition, HDL particles include 2 major particles, lipoprotein ($L_p$) A-I (which is lipid-free HDL and represents 70% of total HDL protein) and $L_pA$-II (about 20% of the total), and 2 minor lipoprotein particles, $L_pE$ and $L_pE$:A-I (**Fig. 3**). The concentration of apoA-I in normal individuals is approximately 1.0 g/L, making it one of the most abundant proteins in human plasma. Virtually all of the apoA-II resides in A-I/A-II HDLs in most people, whereas apoA-I is distributed equally between A-I HDLs and A-I/A-II HDLs. A small proportion of the apoA-I exists in a lipid-free or lipid-poor form. Some HDL particles also contain other minor apolipoproteins such as apoA-IV, apoA-V, apoC-I, apoC-II, apoC-III, apoD, apoJ, and apoL. HDLs also transport several additional proteins, including paraoxonase (PON), cholesteryl ester transfer protein (CETP), lecithin:cholesterol acyltransferase (LCAT), and phospholipid transfer protein (PLTP).

## MECHANISMS OF ANTIATHEROGENIC PROPERTIES OF HDL

Several explanations have been ascribed for the beneficial effects of HDL-C on atherogenesis, particularly its role on reverse cholesterol transport.[18] This process involves the transport of excessive cholesterol from foam macrophages in the arterial wall to HDL-C particles and onto the feces via the liver and bile (**Fig. 4**). The large $HDL_2$ particles promote cholesterol transport through the adenosine triphosphate cassette–binding transporter ABCG1 pathway, whereas the smaller $HDL_3$ particles more efficiently enhance cholesterol efflux through the ABCA1 pathway.[19] Other beneficial effects of cholesterol include antioxidant, antiapoptotic, and antiinflammatory

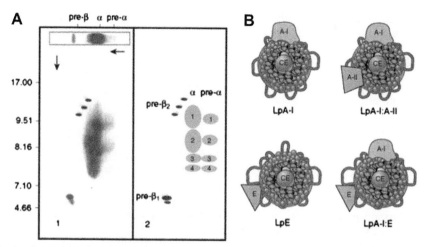

**Fig. 3.** Plasma two-dimensional gel electrophoresis of plasma high-density lipoprotein (HDL) (*A*) and the major HDL particles classified according to apolipoprotein composition (*B*). CE, cholesteryl ester. (*From* Ballantyne CM. Clinical lipidology: a companion to Braunwald's heart disease. Philadelphia: Saunders/Elsevier; 2009. p. 46; with permission.)

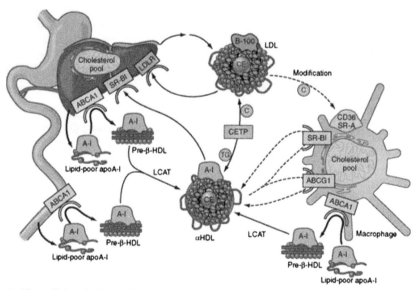

**Fig. 4.** The cellular cholesterol level in the liver, intestine, and macrophage is modulated by HDL. An increased level of cellular cholesterol in the liver, intestine, or macrophage upregulates the level of expression of ATP-binding cassette A1 (ABCA1) and increases cholesterol efflux to the lipid-poor apolipoprotein (apo) A-I with ultimate production of α-HDL following cholesterol esterification by LCAT. Increased intracellular levels of cholesterol also increases the ABCG1 transporter and, in conjunction with scavenger receptor class B type I receptor (SR-BI), increases cholesterol efflux to α-HDL. Cholesterol is transported back to the liver either following transfer to apoB-containing lipoproteins by the CETP or directly to the liver by selective update of HDL-free cholesterol by interaction of HDL with the hepatic SR-BI. A-I, apolipoprotein A-I; LCAT, lecithin:cholesterol acyltransferase. (*From* Ballantyne CM. Clinical lipidology: a companion to Braunwald's heart disease. Philadelphia: Saunders/Elsevier; 2009. p. 49; with permission.)

properties[20]; improved endothelial function by increasing activity of nitric oxide synthase; and anticoagulant effects (**Fig. 5**).[21]

## AGENTS THAT INCREASE HDL-C

In addition to lifestyle changes, such as weight reduction, physical activity, smoking cessation, and moderate alcohol consumption, pharmacologic agents have shown promise in increasing HDL levels. These agents include statins, fibrates, niacin, and CETP inhibitors.

### Statins

Statins have been shown to increase HDL-C levels by about 5% to 10%, with the largest increases occurring usually in those with a low HDL-C and increased triglycerides.[22] There are significant differences in the dose-response curve for increases in HDL-C associated with statin therapy. In general, the maximal HDL-C increases are observed at starting doses or low doses of statins and, in the instance of atorvastatin, there is a reversal of HDL-C increases at higher doses. The mechanism by which statins increase the concentration of HDL-C is unclear. In one meta-analysis of 32,258 patients treated with rosuvastatin, atorvastatin, or simvastatin there was a dose-dependent increase in HDL-C with both rosuvastatin and simvastatin, whereas, for atorvastatin, the increase in HDL-C was inversely related to dose.[22] There was no relationship between statin-induced changes in HDL-C and changes in LDL-C. Pretreatment HDL-C levels were the strongest predictor of statin-induced increase in HDL-C: the lower the pretreatment HDL-C level, the greater the increase in HDL-C after statin therapy. However, in patients with type 2 diabetes, the increase in HDL-C with statin therapy was less than in those without diabetes, even though those in the diabetes group had lower levels of HDL-C.

### Fibrates

Fibrates are associated with only modest changes in HDL-C levels (2%–20%)[23] and could possibly increase LDL-C levels. In one large study, therapy with fenofibrate

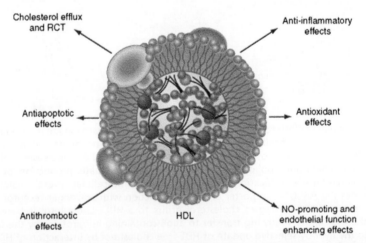

**Fig. 5.** Mechanisms by which HDL may be antiatherogenic. RCT, reverse cholesterol transport. (*From* Ballantyne CM. Clinical lipidology: a companion to Braunwald's heart disease. Philadelphia: Saunders/Elsevier; 2009. p. 545; with permission.)

increased HDL-C levels by less than 2% in patients with diabetes.[24] The beneficial effect of fibrates on cardiovascular outcomes is not attributed to its HDL-C–increasing properties.

## Niacin

Niacin (or vitamin $B_3$) was shown to reduce cholesterol in 1955[25,26] and, until recently, was considered promising for risk reduction because it increases HDL-C levels by as much as 15% to 35% in a dose-dependent manner, and also lowers LDL-C and triglycerides. The Coronary Drug Project, which predated the widespread use of statins, reported that niacin had a beneficial outcome in that it reduced the incidence of all-cause mortality by 9% at the end of 15 years and the incidence of nonfatal myocardial infarction by 27% ($P<.004$) at the end of 5 years.[27] The Coronary Drug Project was a randomized, double-blind, placebo-controlled trial conducted between 1966 and 1974. This trial investigated the effects of 5 lipid-modifying agents (low-dose estrogen, high-dose estrogen, clofibrate, dextrothyroxine, and niacin) in 8341 men (aged 40–64 years) with a history of previous myocardial infarction (MI) and hypercholesterolemia. The low-dose and high-dose estrogen groups and the dextrothyroxine groups were discontinued before the scheduled completion of the study because of adverse side effects. The clofibrate and niacin groups completed the study (total follow-up ranged from 5 to 8.5 years per patient; mean follow-up was 6.2 years). There were 2789 patients in the placebo group and 1119 patients in the niacin group, and the primary end point was total mortality. Total mortality was similar in the 2 groups at 5 years (24.4% with niacin vs 25.4% with placebo, $P$ = not significant). In this study, most patients were not on aspirin, ACE inhibitors, or statin therapy, which is now known to be beneficial in this cohort. A more recent study, the Atherothrombosis Intervention in Metabolic Syndrome with Low HDL/High Triglycerides: Impact on Global Health Outcomes trial (AIM-HIGH), suggests that increasing HDL levels with niacin therapy may not have incremental outcomes benefit to patients with baseline LDL-C levels below 70 mg/dL due to statin treatment.[28] This study was designed with 85% power to show a 25% reduction in the primary end point (a composite of the first event of death from CHD, hospitalization for an acute coronary syndrome, nonfatal MI, ischemic stroke, or symptom-driven coronary or cerebral revascularization), with the addition of 1.5 to 2 g of niacin per day in patients more than 45 years of age with known cardiovascular disease and dyslipidemia. Despite attaining desirable levels of HDL cholesterol (an increase of 25%), LDL cholesterol (a decrease of 12%), and triglycerides (a decrease of 29%) with niacin therapy, there was no reduction in the incidence of the primary composite end point, and it did not show any clinical benefit overall or in a major subgroup. The data and safety monitoring board stopped the clinical trial prematurely because the boundary for futility had been crossed, and an unexpectedly higher number of ischemic strokes were observed in patients assigned to niacin. These results do not support the addition of niacin to statin therapy in patients who have achieved LDL goals. In addition, the possible risk of increased risk of ischemic stroke with niacin and the flushing side effects of niacin make it particularly unattractive for routine risk reduction. However, niacin may have a role in statin-intolerant patients. HPS2-THRIVE (Heart Protection Study2-Treatment of HDL to Reduce the Incidence of Vascular Events), a larger ongoing clinical trial, is currently evaluating the role of niacin and should give the final answer on cardiovascular outcomes.

## CETP Inhibitors

CETP is a plasma protein that facilitates the transfer of cholesteryl esters from HDL-C to LDL-C and triglycerides. CETP is not found in most species, but occurs in humans, nonhuman primates, and rabbits, and these are the species that are more susceptible to development of atherosclerotic disease. Inhibition of CETP results in increased HDL-C levels (including apolipoprotein A1 levels) and some reductions in LDL-C levels (including apoB levels). Agents belonging to this class include ancetrapib,[29] dalcetrapib,[30-32] evacetrapib,[33] and torcetrapib. One suggested limitation of these agents is whether the larger cholesterol-rich HDL particles, formed as a result of their inhibition, are able to function effectively in reverse cholesterol transport. However, in vitro studies have suggested that HDL particles formed as a result of inhibition with either torcetrapib or anacetrapib have normal, or possibly even enhanced, ability to promote cholesterol efflux for macrophages.[34-36] The use of CETP inhibitors in clinical trials has currently not met the promise because of side effects or lack of incremental benefit on cardiovascular outcomes, or both. In the Investigation of Lipid Level Management to Understand its Impact in Atherosclerotic Events (ILLUMINATE) trial, torcetrapib was found to be associated with increased cardiovascular events, increased overall mortality,[37] increases in blood pressure, increase in circulating aldosterone levels, and altered serum electrolytes. Torcetrapib also results in increased synthesis of both aldosterone and cortisol levels in adrenal cortical cells.[38,39] Unlike torcetrapib, none of the other CETP inhibitors have been shown to affect blood pressure, serum aldosterone levels, or electrolytes. A more recent trial evaluating the role of evacetrapib used as monotherapy or in combination with statins showed a 132% relative increase in HDL-C, a 40% decrease in LDL-C levels with no changes in blood pressure, serum aldosterone levels, or liver function tests.[33] Promising results regarding dalcetrapib have been reported in phase 2 studies[30-32] and a large phase 3 clinical trial is currently ongoing and results are awaited.[40] Similarly, anacetrapib studies have produced early reports of promising safety and efficacy,[29,41-43] and a phase 3 clinical trial has started enrolling.

## SUMMARY

An inverse relationship between the plasma concentration of HDL-C and the risk of having a cardiovascular event has been shown in several epidemiologic studies. It is likely that this relationship is causal because HDL has several intrinsic properties that can potentially reverse atherosclerosis (see **Fig. 5**). Despite several animal studies showing that increasing HDL with pharmacologic agents is beneficial for atherosclerosis, this has not been conclusively shown in humans. Several clinical trials evaluating various pharmacologic agents are ongoing and their results are awaited. Pharmacotherapy altering lipid profiles may have reached its potential for risk reduction, and adding agents to increase the good cholesterol to reduce risk is associated with minimal incremental outcome benefits; trying to achieve perfection with pharmacotherapy is possibly the enemy of good (ie, a healthy lifestyle).[44] Until there are more data showing the beneficial effects of pharmacotherapy, patients with low HDL should be advised to change their lifestyle, including smoking cessation, weight reduction, and regular exercise.

## REFERENCES

1. Baliga RR, Cannon CP. Dyslipidemia. Oxford (UK): Oxford University Press; 2011.
2. Baliga RR. Statin prescribing guide. New York: Oxford University Press; 2009.
3. Baigent C, Blackwell L, Emberson J, et al. Efficacy and safety of more intensive lowering of LDL cholesterol: a meta-analysis of data from 170,000 participants in 26 randomised trials. Lancet 2010;376(9753):1670-81.

4. Baigent C, Keech A, Kearney PM, et al. Efficacy and safety of cholesterol-lowering treatment: prospective meta-analysis of data from 90,056 participants in 14 randomised trials of statins. Lancet 2005;366(9493):1267–78.

5. Pedersen TR, Faergeman O, Kastelein JJ, et al. High-dose atorvastatin vs usual-dose simvastatin for secondary prevention after myocardial infarction: the IDEAL study: a randomized controlled trial. JAMA 2005;294(19):2437–45.

6. LaRosa JC, Grundy SM, Waters DD, et al. Intensive lipid lowering with atorvastatin in patients with stable coronary disease. N Engl J Med 2005;352(14):1425–35.

7. Castelli WP, Garrison RJ, Wilson PW, et al. Incidence of coronary heart disease and lipoprotein cholesterol levels. The Framingham Study. JAMA 1986;256(20):2835–8.

8. Gordon T, Castelli WP, Hjortland MC, et al. High density lipoprotein as a protective factor against coronary heart disease. The Framingham Study. Am J Med 1977;62(5):707–14.

9. Alsheikh-Ali AA, Abjourjaily HM, Stanek E, et al. Increases in HDL-cholesterol are the strongest predictors of risk reduction in lipid intervention trials. American Heart Association Scientific Sessions. New Orleans (LA), November 7–10, 2004.

10. Kannel WB. High-density lipoproteins: epidemiologic profile and risks of coronary artery disease. Am J Cardiol 1983;52(4):9B–12B.

11. Gordon DJ, Probstfield JL, Garrison RJ, et al. High-density lipoprotein cholesterol and cardiovascular disease. Four prospective American studies. Circulation 1989;79(1):8–15.

12. Castelli WP. Cholesterol and lipids in the risk of coronary artery disease–the Framingham Heart Study. Can J Cardiol 1988;4(Suppl A):5A–10A.

13. Packard CJ, Ford I, Robertson M, et al. Plasma lipoproteins and apolipoproteins as predictors of cardiovascular risk and treatment benefit in the PROspective Study of Pravastatin in the Elderly at Risk (PROSPER). Circulation 2005;112(20):3058–65.

14. Nicholls SJ, Ballantyne CM, Barter PJ, et al. Effect of two intensive statin regimens on progression of coronary disease. N Engl J Med 2011;365(22):2078–87.

15. Barter P, Gotto AM, LaRosa JC, et al. HDL cholesterol, very low levels of LDL cholesterol, and cardiovascular events. N Engl J Med 2007;357(13):1301–10.

16. Ford ES, Giles WH, Dietz WH. Prevalence of the metabolic syndrome among US adults: findings from the third National Health and Nutrition Examination Survey. JAMA 2002;287(3):356–9.

17. Rye KA, Clay MA, Barter PJ. Remodelling of high density lipoproteins by plasma factors. Atherosclerosis 1999;145(2):227–38.

18. von Eckardstein A, Nofer JR, Assmann G. High density lipoproteins and arteriosclerosis. Role of cholesterol efflux and reverse cholesterol transport. Arterioscler Thromb Vasc Biol 2001;21(1):13–27.

19. Tall AR. Role of ABCA1 in cellular cholesterol efflux and reverse cholesterol transport. Arterioscler Thromb Vasc Biol 2003;23(5):710–1.

20. Barter PJ, Nicholls S, Rye KA, et al. Antiinflammatory properties of HDL. Circ Res 2004;95(8):764–72.

21. Mineo C, Deguchi H, Griffin JH, et al. Endothelial and antithrombotic actions of HDL. Circ Res 2006;98(11):1352–64.

22. Barter PJ, Brandrup-Wognsen G, Palmer MK, et al. Effect of statins on HDL-C: a complex process unrelated to changes in LDL-C: analysis of the VOYAGER Database. J Lipid Res 2010;51(6):1546–53.

23. Stamler JA, The Coronary Drug Project Research Group. Clofibrate and niacin in coronary heart disease. JAMA 1975;231(4):360–81.

24. Keech A, Simes RJ, Barter P, et al. Effects of long-term fenofibrate therapy on cardiovascular events in 9795 people with type 2 diabetes mellitus (the FIELD study): randomised controlled trial. Lancet 2005;366(9500):1849–61.

25. Altschul R, Hoffer A, Stephen JD. Influence of nicotinic acid on serum cholesterol in man. Arch Biochem Biophys 1955;54(2):558–9.

26. Giugliano RP. Niacin at 56 years of age–time for an early retirement? N Engl J Med 2011;365(24):2318–20.

27. Canner PL, Berge KG, Wenger NK, et al. Fifteen year mortality in Coronary Drug Project patients: long-term benefit with niacin. J Am Coll Cardiol 1986;8(6):1245–55.

28. Boden WE, Probstfield JL, Anderson T, et al. Niacin in patients with low HDL cholesterol levels receiving intensive statin therapy. N Engl J Med 2011;365(24):2255–67.

29. Cannon CP, Shah S, Dansky HM, et al. Safety of anacetrapib in patients with or at high risk for coronary heart disease. N Engl J Med 2010;363(25):2406–15.

30. Kastelein JJ, Duivenvoorden R, Deanfield J, et al. Rationale and design of dal-VESSEL: a study to assess the safety and efficacy of dalcetrapib on endothelial function using brachial artery flow-mediated vasodilatation. Curr Med Res Opin 2011;27(1):141–50.

31. Fayad ZA, Mani V, Woodward M, et al. Safety and efficacy of dalcetrapib on atherosclerotic disease using novel non-invasive multimodality imaging (dal-PLAQUE): a randomised clinical trial. Lancet 2011;378(9802):1547–59.

32. Stein EA, Roth EM, Rhyne JM, et al. Safety and tolerability of dalcetrapib (RO4607381/JTT-705): results from a 48-week trial. Eur Heart J 2010;31(4):480–8.

33. Nicholls SJ, Brewer HB, Kastelein JJ, et al. Effects of the CETP inhibitor evacetrapib administered as monotherapy or in combination with statins on HDL and LDL cholesterol: a randomized controlled trial. JAMA 2011;306(19):2099–109.

34. Yvan-Charvet L, Kling J, Pagler T, et al. Cholesterol efflux potential and antiinflammatory properties of high-density lipoprotein after treatment with niacin or anacetrapib. Arterioscler Thromb Vasc Biol 2010;30(7):1430–8.

35. Yvan-Charvet L, Matsuura F, Wang N, et al. Inhibition of cholesteryl ester transfer protein by torcetrapib modestly increases macrophage cholesterol efflux to HDL. Arterioscler Thromb Vasc Biol 2007;27(5):1132–8.

36. Matsuura F, Wang N, Chen W, et al. HDL from CETP-deficient subjects shows enhanced ability to promote cholesterol efflux from macrophages in an apoE- and ABCG1-dependent pathway. J Clin Invest 2006;116(5):1435–42.

37. Barter PJ, Caulfield M, Eriksson M, et al. Effects of torcetrapib in patients at high risk for coronary events. N Engl J Med 2007;357(21):2109–22.

38. Forrest MJ, Bloomfield D, Briscoe RJ, et al. Torcetrapib-induced blood pressure elevation is independent of CETP inhibition and is accompanied by increased circulating levels of aldosterone. Br J Pharmacol 2008;154(7):1465–73.

39. Stroes ES, Nierman MC, Meulenberg JJ, et al. Intramuscular administration of AAV1-lipoprotein lipase S447X lowers triglycerides in lipoprotein lipase-deficient patients. Arterioscler Thromb Vasc Biol 2008;28(12):2303–4.

40. Schwartz GG, Olsson AG, Ballantyne CM, et al. Rationale and design of the dal-OUTCOMES trial: efficacy and safety of dalcetrapib in patients with recent acute coronary syndrome. Am Heart J 2009;158(6):896–901, e3.

41. Krishna R, Anderson MS, Bergman AJ, et al. Effect of the cholesteryl ester transfer protein inhibitor, anacetrapib, on lipoproteins in patients with dyslipidaemia and on 24-h ambulatory blood pressure in healthy individuals: two double-blind, randomised placebo-controlled phase I studies. Lancet 2007;370(9603):1907–14.

42. Dansky HM, Bloomfield D, Gibbons P, et al. Efficacy and safety after cessation of treatment with the cholesteryl ester transfer protein inhibitor anacetrapib (MK-0859) in patients with primary hypercholesterolemia or mixed hyperlipidemia. Am Heart J 2011;162(4):708–16.
43. Bloomfield D, Carlson GL, Sapre A, et al. Efficacy and safety of the cholesteryl ester transfer protein inhibitor anacetrapib as monotherapy and coadministered with atorvastatin in dyslipidemic patients. Am Heart J 2009;157(2):352–60, e2.
44. Ben-Shahar T. The pursuit of perfect: how to stop chasing perfection and start living a richer, happier life. New York: McGraw-Hill; 2009.

# Triglycerides: How Much Credit Do They Deserve?

Payal Kohli, MD*, Christopher P. Cannon, MD

**KEYWORDS**

- Hypertriglyceridemia • Dyslipidemia • Statin
- Metabolic syndrome • Diabetes

Triglycerides (TGs) have long been an under-recognized member of the lipid family, and the relationship between hypertriglyceridemia and atherosclerosis continues to remain the subject of intense debate. Whether high levels of TGs have a causal relationship to coronary artery disease (CAD) or are merely biomarkers of concurrent risk factors that lead to CAD is still not firmly established.[1] However, with the rising incidence of atherogenic dyslipidemia, diabetes mellitus, and the metabolic syndrome,[2] TGs are now attracting attention as predictors of risk as well as targets for primary and secondary prevention in patients with metabolic syndrome, diabetes mellitus, and coronary heart disease. Although statin therapy has significantly decreased the disease burden of coronary heart disease in the past decade, residual cardiovascular risk still persists[3] and may be attributed to underlying atherogenic dyslipidemias.[4] In particular, hypertriglyceridemia has been identified as a potential key mediator of atherosclerosis.

## PREVALENCE AND DEFINITION

Hypertriglyceridemia is one of the most common dyslipidemias in the population today[5] and can be defined based on population distributions. Although there is variability among racial groups, the following cutoffs are broadly applied: In general, normal levels are considered less than 150 mg/dL (1.7 mmol/L), borderline high is defined as 150 to 199 mg/dL (1.7–2.2 mmol/L), high is defined as 200 to 499 mg/dL (2.3–5.6 mmol/L), and very high levels are greater than or equal to 500 mg/dL (≥5.7 mmol/L). In the United States, the National Health and Nutrition Examination Surveys, from 1999 to 2004, found that the percentage of adults with elevated TGs are as follows: borderline high (33%), high (18%), and very high (1.7%).[6] Within distinct ethnic

Conflicts of interest: The authors have no conflicts of interest to disclose.
TIMI Study Group, Cardiovascular Division, Department of Medicine, Brigham & Women's Hospital, 350 Longwood Avenue, 1st Floor, Boston, MA 02115, USA
* Corresponding author.
E-mail address: pkohli@partners.org

Med Clin N Am 96 (2012) 39–55
doi:10.1016/j.mcna.2011.11.006
0025-7125/12/$ – see front matter © 2012 Elsevier Inc. All rights reserved.

medical.theclinics.com

groups, Mexican Americans have the highest levels (34.9%), followed by non-Hispanic whites (33%) and blacks (15.6%).[2]

## TG PHYSIOLOGY AND CAUSES OF ELEVATED TGS

Before reviewing the link between TG and CAD, it is prudent to review normal lipoprotein metabolism. Lipoproteins are complexes that transport proteins and lipids in plasma.[2] All circulating lipoproteins are made up of lipids that compose the core, including TGs and cholesterol esters, surface phospholipids, small amounts of free cholesterol, and one or more apolipoproteins.[7] Apolipoproteins are surface proteins on lipoproteins that participate in regulation, signaling and solubilization of lipoproteins. Blood levels of these molecules are regulated by homeostatic mechanisms that balance the rates of secretion from the intestines and liver as well as the rates of catabolism.[8] Hypertriglyceridemia often occurs in patients with diabetes mellitus and the metabolic syndrome and can result from excess production of TGs by hepatocytes or decreased catabolism of TG-rich lipoproteins (**Fig. 1**).[9,10] For example, in patients with insulin resistance, increased secretion of very low-density lipoprotein (VLDL) TGs and TG-rich lipoproteins (TRLs) from the intestines has been proposed as a mechanistic explanation for hypertriglyceridemia.[8] Furthermore, in these patients, hepatic secretion of apolipoprotein C-III (apoC-III) is increased, which delays the catabolism of TRLs, resulting in elevated serum concentrations. In addition, high TGs have been implicated in remodeling of the low-density lipoprotein (LDL) and high-density lipoprotein (HDL) particles, making them smaller and denser and enriching them with TGs.[8,11] In patients with metabolic syndrome, the increased mass of adipose tissue is unable to efficiently sequester free fatty acids, leading to increased conversion of fatty acids to TGs, hepatic steatosis, and overproduction of VLDL particles.[9] Furthermore, it seems that visceral adiposity exposes the liver to higher levels of circulating free fatty acids and increases the efflux of VLDLs, leading to a more severe elevation in TG concentration, when compared with subcutaneous adiposity.[12,13]

## GENETIC STUDIES IN HYPERTRIGLYCERIDEMIA

In addition to acquired causes of hypertriglyceridemia, there are several genetic causes. Familial hypertriglyceridemia, also known as type IV hyperlipoproteinemia, has a prevalence of 1% to 2% and provides clues into the genetic basis for elevated TGs. In this disorder, plasma TG, VLDL cholesterol, and VLDL TGs are moderately to markedly elevated and LDL and HDL levels are usually low.[14] Patients with this disorder are very sensitive to alcohol and caloric and carbohydrate intake, which stimulates production of TGs. A multigenic inheritance is theorized because of the degree of clinical heterogeneity observed.[14] Similarly, type V hyperlipidemia, a rare disorder, which results in overproduction levels of VLDL and chylomicrons, is thought to be multifactorial, linked to environmental exposures, and genetically heterogeneous.[2] Sarwar and colleagues[15] identified a regulatory variant (-1131T>C) in the promoter region of the APOA5 gene that is related, in a dose-dependent fashion, to TG concentrations and to the risk of coronary heart disease. In their large study of 20,842 patients with coronary heart disease and 35,206 controls, they concluded that the risk of coronary heart disease is approximately 18% higher per C allele inherited and that this risk may be mediated, in part, via higher VLDL concentrations and smaller HDL particle size.[15]

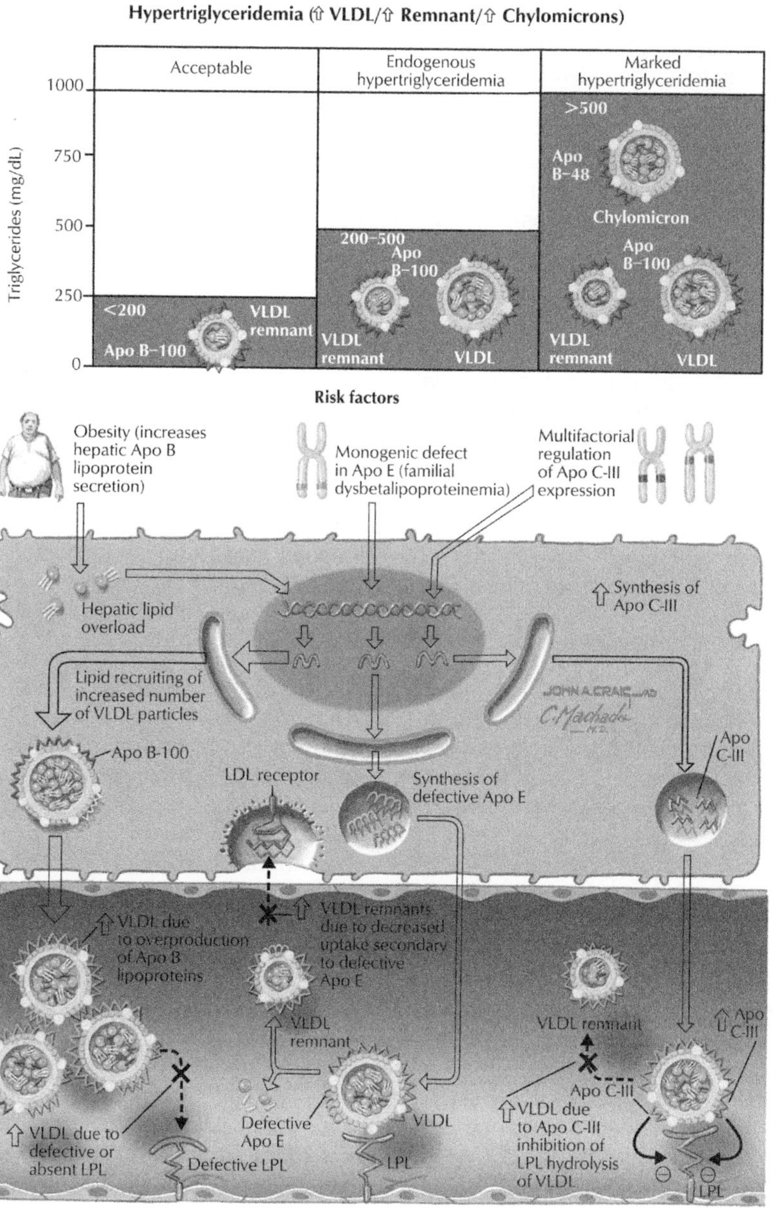

Fig. 1. Metabolism of TGs and physiologic mechanisms of hypertriglyceridemia. Apo, apolipoprotein; LDL, low density lipoprotein; LPL, lipoprotein lipase; VLDL, very low density lipoprotein. (Netter illustration from netterimages.com. © Elsevier Inc. All rights reserved.)

## MEASURING TGS

Several challenges exist in measuring and following this lipid molecule. Firstly, its distribution in serum is markedly skewed and requires log transformation to normalize.[2] At high levels, checking serum concentration of TGs is unreliable because the ratio of TGs to cholesterol esters increases in VLDL particles. Therefore, mathematical calculations become inaccurate.[16] Secondly, lipoprotein metabolism is intricately linked and elevations in TGs can be confounded by changes in HDL, LDL, VLDL, and total cholesterol. There seems to be a strong inverse relationship between TG concentration and HDL cholesterol (HDL-C) and apolipoprotein A-1 (apoA-1).[2] Thirdly, there is high intra-individual variability, and this variability is amplified at high TG concentrations,[2] making this a less-stable parameter to follow as compared to HDL and LDL. Furthermore, nonlipid risk factors for atherosclerosis, such as obesity, diabetes, hypertension, and smoking, are highly correlated with increased TGs, and these factors can independently confer risk for coronary heart disease.[17]

## BIOLOGIC ROLE OF TGS IN CAD

Despite these confounders, however, TGs have been directly implicated in microvascular and macrovascular endothelial damage via several distinct mechanisms, including increased inflammation, foam cell formation, smooth muscle cell toxicity oxidative stress, accelerated senescence, and impaired vascular repair.[18,19] Several experimental studies have suggested that HDL and LDL particles that are enriched in TGs may be more likely to undergo oxidative modification[20,21] and may be more dysfunctional[22,23] and harmful to endothelial cells than their less-dense counterparts. Although the biologic mechanisms are well defined, clinical and epidemiologic data have yielded controversial results regarding the independent risk conferred by TGs.

## EVIDENCE FOR TGS AS AN INDEPENDENT RISK FACTOR FOR CAD

The finding that patients with premature CAD have an 80% to 88% incidence of hypertriglyceridemia compared with 40% to 48% in age-matched controls without CAD[24,25] has established the relationship between hypertriglyceridemia and atherosclerosis. The debate regarding association versus causality began in 1980, when an epidemiologic analyses published in the *New England Journal of Medicine* did not identify TGs as an independent risk factor and concluded that the evidence for a casual relationship was "meager."[1] This lack of association was attributed to the presence of several confounding variables, such as other lipids and nonlipid risk factors for obesity, hypertension, diabetes, and cigarette smoking, that correlate with hypertriglyceridemia[1,17]; the predictive capacity of TGs was weakened after adjustment for covariates, such as plasma glucose and HDL-C.[26]

However, the interest in TGs as coronary risk factors reemerged in the 1990s when a series of studies demonstrated that elevated TGs may indeed confer *independent* CAD risk. In 1996, the results of a meta-analysis of 17 prospective population-based studies concluded that increase in plasma TG concentrations was an *independent* risk factor for the development of CAD and that this effect was magnified in women compared with men.[27] These conclusions were similar to another pooled analyses in the Asia-Pacific region.[28] In younger patients, lowering TG levels led to a decrease in the risk of incident CAD.[29] A large meta-analysis of 262,525 patients suggested a hazard ratio (HR) of 1.72 (95% confidence interval [CI] 156.0–1.90) for the risk of coronary heart disease between patients in the highest and lowest quartiles of TGs.[30] These results continued to spark intense discussion regarding the importance and the role of these lipid molecules in the pathogenesis of heart disease and the debate surged on.

More recently, several studies have identified TGs as a risk factor for the development of CAD and major adverse cardiovascular events (**Fig. 2**).[30–32] In a matched case-control study of patients from Brigham & Women's Hospital in Boston, Massachusetts, 170 subjects (those who developed incident CAD) and 175 controls (those

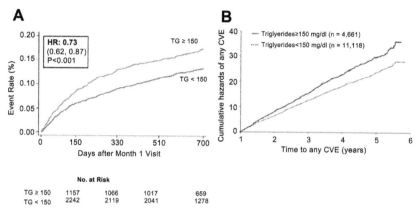

**Fig. 2.** Cardiovascular events stratified by on-treatment TGs greater than or equal to 150 mg/dL or less than 150 mg/dL. (*A*) Kaplan-Meier event rate for composite endpoint (death, myocardial infarction, and recurrent ACS), starting at 30 days until 2 years of follow-up, is significantly lower (HR 0.73, 95% CI 0.62–1.87, *P*<.001) for patients with lower on-treatment TGs. (*B*) Cumulative risk of any cardiovascular event in patients enrolled in the TNT or IDEAL studies is decreased in patients with TGs less than 150 mg/dL (n = 11,118) compared with TGs greater than or equal to 150 mg/dL (n = 4661). CVE, cardiovascular event. (*From* (*A*) Miller M, Cannon CP, Murphy SA, et al. Impact of triglyceride levels beyond low-density lipoprotein cholesterol after acute coronary syndrome in the PROVE IT-TIMI 22 trial. J AmColl Cardiol 2008;51(7):724–30; with permission; and (*B*) Faergeman O, Holme I, Fayyad R, et al. Plasma triglycerides and cardiovascular events in the Treating to New Targets and Incremental Decrease in End-Points through Aggressive Lipid Lowering trials of statins in patients with coronary artery disease. Am J Cardiol 2009;104(4):459–63; with permission.)

without incident CAD) were studied to determine the residual risk of TGs in patients with LDL less than 130 mg/dL. HDL values were variable. The investigators concluded that the odds of CAD increased by approximately 20% per 23 mg/dL increase in TGs and by 40% per 7.5 mg/dL decrease in HDL cholesterol and the combination was synergistic to increase the odds ratio to 10× in those patients with the highest TGs and lowest HDL.[30] The Helsinki Heart study, a 5-year randomized study of dyslipidemia in 4081 men, found that elevated TGs were prognostic for coronary heart disease risk, especially when used in combination with HDL and LDL.[33] In the Pravastatin or Atorvastatin Evaluation and Infection Therapy–Thrombolysis in Myocardial Infarction 22 (PROVE-IT) Thrombolysis in Myocardial Infarction (TIMI)-22 cohort, which analyzed patients with recent acute coronary syndrome (ACS), on-treatment TGs greater than 150 mg/dL were *independently* associated with a higher risk of recurrent coronary events (death, myocardial infarction [MI], and recurrent ACS) after adjustment for LDL-C, non–high-density lipoprotein cholesterol, and other covariates (**Fig. 3**).[32] In these patients with ACS, despite achieving target LDL-C values (<70 mg/dL), each 10 mg/dL decrease in on-treatment TGs resulted in a lowering of the composite endpoint of death, MI, or recurrent stroke by 1.6% (*P*<.001) or 1.4% (when adjusted for LDL-C and other covariates, *P* = .01).

There are, however, studies in which TGs lose significance as a predictive biomarker when a multivariable model is completely adjusted for covariates. The substudy of the Incremental Decrease in End Points through Aggressive Lipid Lowering (IDEAL) and Treating to New Targets (TNT) parent trials examined this risk relationship in patients with stable CAD. After adjusting for age, gender, and study, the risk of cardiovascular events increased with increasing TGs, with patients in the highest

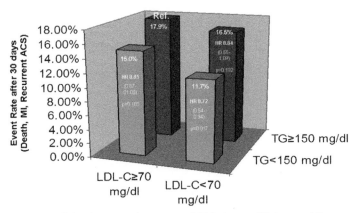

**Fig. 3.** Highest rate of death, MI, and recurrent ACS between 30 days and 2 years of follow-up is seen in patients with LDL-C greater than or equal to 70 mg/dL and TG greater than or equal to 150 mg/dL. This model is adjusted for age, gender, low HDL, smoking, hypertension, diabetes, obesity, prior statin therapy, prior ACS, peripheral vascular disease, and treatment effect. Ref., referent group. (*Data from* Miller M, Cannon CP, Murphy SA, et al. Impact of triglyceride levels beyond low-density lipoprotein cholesterol after acute coronary syndrome in the PROVE IT-TIMI 22 trial. J Am Coll Cardiol 2008;51(7):724–30.)

quintile having a 63% higher risk of events (HR 1.46–1.81) after the first year of the trial. The predictive effect of TGs was dampened when HDL-C and apoB/apoAI were introduced into the model and was completely eliminated when diabetes, body mass index, glucose, hypertension, and smoking were added.[31] The same trend was seen in patients who were at target LDL-C concentrations (<100 mg/dL).

In 2003, the National Cholesterol Education Program (NCEP) expert panel (Adult Treatment Panel III [ATP III]) revised its guidelines and identified non–HDL-C (total cholesterol minus HDL cholesterol) as a secondary target in patients with TG greater than 200 mg/dL, after adequate LDL control.

## NONPHARMACOLOGIC AND PHARMACOLOGIC TREATMENT OF HYPERTRIGLYCERIDEMIA

Following the release of the ATP III guidelines and in the face of mounting evidence for the potential benefit associated with lowering TGs, treatment of hypertriglyceridemia with nonpharmacologic and pharmacologic means has become common in patients who have CAD or are at risk for premature atherosclerosis. The evidence in favor of treatment of severe hypertriglyceridemia (>1000–1500 mg/dL or 11.3–16.9 mmol/L) is convincing,[34,35] but randomized controlled trial data regarding treatment of mild to moderate hypertriglyceridemia has not revealed consistent results.[36] Recently in April 2011, however, the American Heart Association issued a scientific statement indicating that the optimal fasting TG concentration may be less than 100 mg/dL (with nonfasting concentrations <200 mg/dL), although it cautioned against using these numbers as therapeutic targets for drugs, recommending instead nonpharmacologic and therapeutic lifestyle changes as first-line interventions.[2]

Overall, the combination of lifestyle changes, including diet, exercise, and weight loss, can result in a potent up to 50% decrease in TG concentrations.[2] Among the many lifestyle modifications recommended, weight loss, even if it is moderate, results in an approximately 22% decrease in TGs; an approximately 9% increase in HDL;

a decrease in small, dense LDL particles by up to 40%[37]; and a decreased incidence of coronary disease, diabetes mellitus, and associated TG abnormalities.[38–40] The rate of change in TGs is directly related to the degree of weight loss. In association with weight loss, regular aerobic exercise of moderate intensity (~4 h/wk) can result in a decrease in intra-abdominal adiposity and an increase in HDL cholesterol and concurrent decrease in TG, although a direct dose-response relationship has not yet been established.[41–43] Dietary recommendations suggest a balanced caloric intake with a diet rich in fruits and vegetables, whole grains, and fiber and consumption of oily fish.[39,40] Because diets low in fat and high in carbohydrates result in reduction in both LDL and HDL cholesterol, current recommendations suggest replacing saturated fat with complex carbohydrates and unsaturated fats[39–41] and avoiding simple sugars, which have been associated with postprandial hypertriglyceridemia.[44] Modest alcohol intake, cessation of cigarette smoking, and ω-3 supplementation have been associated with decreases in VLDL TG levels and, interestingly, modest caffeine intake has also been linked to lower TG concentration.[41,45]

Although lifestyle modifications are remarkably effective in lowering and maintaining TG concentrations, pharmacologic treatment is often required in select high-risk patients (**Table 1**).[46] Mechanistically, effective therapies for hypertriglyceridemia target kinetic defects in the anabolism and catabolism of TGs, by decreasing hepatic secretion of VLDL, apoB, and TGs, increasing transfer of apoB from VLDL to LDL, or increasing clearance of apoB-containing lipoproteins.[9]

Statin monotherapy is considered the first-line therapy primarily because of its potent effects on lowering LDL-cholesterol and apoB.[9,47] Its ability to lower TGs is directly proportional to its efficacy in lowering LDL,[9] but studies have cited 5% to 30% reduction in TG concentration.[32,47,48] Potent statins, such as rosuvastatin, decrease production of LDL-apoB-100 and decrease the breakdown of HDL-apoAl, but this mechanism is not consistently seen with lower potency statins that are, nevertheless, effective in lowering TGs.[9,46] This finding suggests that modulation of partitioning of TGs in the liver may be an additional mechanism by which statins can lower serum TG concentrations. Although statins have consistently shown a reduction in cardiovascular events,[49,50] with an average of 20% to 25% reduction in events per 1 mmol/L reduction in LDL cholesterol,[3] high TGs continue to confer risk.[30] On a background of intensive statin therapy, TG less than 150 mg/dL are independently associated with a lower risk of recurrent coronary events even in the setting of low LDL concentrations (see **Fig. 2**A).[32]

Statins can lower TG concentration, but their effect is dose dependent. Standard dose statin therapy decreases TGs by 8% and intensive therapy reduces TGs by an additional 20% to 30%.[48] Ezetimibe decreases LDL by 10% to 20% and has minimal effects on TGs and HDL cholesterol.[9] Fibrates continue to be one of the more potent agents for decreasing plasma TGs (18%–45%) and can also decrease LDL cholesterol (up to 20%) and raise HDL (up to 20%), making them a popular choice for treatment of dyslipidemias.[51–53] By acting as agonists of the peroxisome proliferator–activated receptor-α (PPAR-α), fibrates transcriptionally regulate genes that are responsible for lipid metabolism and endothelial function.[54,55] They were introduced in Europe more than 35 years ago because of dramatic effects on lipid profiles. Despite their efficacy on lipid parameters, however, their clinical benefit remains uncertain.[56] Two randomized controlled trials that were conducted before widespread use of statins, one of primary prevention in middle-aged men[57] and the other of secondary prevention in patients with CAD with low HDL cholesterol,[58] demonstrated improvement in cardiovascular outcomes of patients treated with gemfibrozil compared with placebo. However, subsequent trials using different fibrates (bezafibrate and fenofibrate) have

**Table 1**
Nonpharmacologic and pharmacologic management of hypertriglyceridemia

| | Percentage Reduction in TGs | Mechanisms of Action | Recommendations | Relevant Studies |
|---|---|---|---|---|
| Lifestyle Modification | — | -Affects partitioning of TGs in liver | — | — |
| Diet | 10%–20% | -Decreased incidence of diabetic dyslipidemia and metabolic syndrome | -Decrease dietary fat<br>-Replace saturated fat with monounsaturated/polyunsaturated fat<br>-Avoid simple carbohydrates | Miller et al,[2] Havel[44] |
| Exercise[a]/Weight Loss | 20% (with weight loss of 5%–10%) OR 1.9% per kilogram of weight lost | -Decreased incidence of diabetic dyslipidemia and metabolic syndrome/intra-abdominal fat<br>-Decreased number of small, dense LDL particles | -Daily walking or high-frequency aerobic exercise (4 times/wk) | Purnell et al,[37] Knowler et al,[38] Lichtenstein et al,[39] Tuomilehto et al,[76] Van Gaal et al,[77] Anderson & Konz,[78] Dattilo & Kris-Etherton[79] |
| Cessation of Cigarette Smoking | Unknown | -Decreased endothelial dysfunction | — | Brunzell[41] |
| Cessation of Alcohol Intake | 5%–10% per ounce decreased | -Decreased cardiovascular risk | -Alcohol in moderation is permitted except in patients with severe hypertriglyceridemia (>2000 mg/dL) | Taskinen,[10] Erkelens & Brunzell,[80] Rimm et al[81] |
| **Medication Class** | | | | |
| Statins | 20%–30% (high-dose statins) | -Decrease hepatic output of VLDL apoB<br>-Decrease catabolism of HDL-apoAI-particles | Dose depends on agent used | Miller et al,[32] Grundy et al,[47] Gibson et al,[48] Cannon et al,[82] Baigent et al[83] |

| | | | | |
|---|---|---|---|---|
| Fibrates | 18%–45% | -Agonists of PPAR-α to mediate transcriptional regulation of lipid metabolism and endothelial function | -Gemfibrozil, 600 mg twice/d<br>-Fenofibrate, 145 mg once/d | Ginsberg et al,[51] Jun et al,[52] Keech et al[53] |
| Niacin | 17%–26% (dose dependent) | -Decreases tissue lipolysis and flux of FFAs to the liver<br>-Direct inhibition of TG synthesis<br>-Decreased VLDL production | 1500–2000 mg once/d (sustained release formulation) | Taylor et al,[66] "Clofibrate and Niacin in Coronary Heart Disease"[84] |
| Ezetimibe | Minor | -Inhibits cholesterol absorption of TGs<br>-Increases catabolism of LDL-C | 10 mg | Goldberg et al[85] |
| ω-3 fatty acid | Dose dependent: approximately 5%–10% per 1g EPA/DHA (up to 25%–30% with 4 g/d of ω-3 PUFAs) | -Improve TG metabolism via transcriptional changes of genes involved in lipogenesis and fatty acid oxidation<br>-Increases conversion of VLDL to LDL<br>-Decrease VLDL secretion | 2–4 g of EPA+DHA | "Dietary Supplementation with n-3 Polyunsaturated Fatty Acids..."[86] Yokoyama et al,[87] Balk et al,[88] Harris[89] |

*Abbreviations:* DHA, docosahexaenoic acid; EPA, eicosapentaenoic acid; FFA, free fatty acid; PPAR-α, peroxisome proliferator–activated receptor-α; PUFAs, polyunsaturated fatty acids.

[a] Effects of exercise of TGs depend on baseline TGs, level and duration of activity, and caloric expenditure.

failed to validate these results,[51,53,59] and select early studies with clofibrate revealed a higher incidence of noncoronary deaths. These results were not confirmed with fenofibrate.[51,53]

Several studies have attempted to answer the question of whether diabetic patients with CAD, who theoretically have a higher risk of worse outcomes from hypertriglyceridemia compared with the baseline population,[51] would benefit from fibrates or combination therapy with statins and fibrates. Data from the Fenofibrate Intervention in Event Lowering in Diabetes (FIELD) study established that the greatest benefit of TG reduction was seen in patients with underlying atherogenic or diabetic dyslipidemia (TG $\geq$2.3 mmol/L, HDL-C <1 mmol/L for men and <1.3 mmol/L for women).[60] There was a 27% relative risk reduction in these patients with a number needed to treat of 23 patients for 5 years to avoid one cardiovascular event. The Action to Control Cardiovascular Risk in Diabetes-Lipid (ACCORD-Lipid) study was a substudy of the parent trial designed to assess the benefit of a statin plus fenofibrate versus statin alone in patients with diabetes with CAD risk factors and excellent glycemic and blood pressure control. This trial randomized 5,518 patients who had already achieved their LDL-C targets. After a mean of 4.7 years of follow-up, fenofibrate plus statin did not decrease the primary endpoint (fatal cardiovascular events, nonfatal MI, or nonfatal stroke) despite a significant decrease in plasma TGs (-22.2% for fibrate plus statin vs -8.7% for statin alone) and an increase in HDL-C (+8.44% vs +6.0% with simvastatin alone).[51] A subgroup analysis, which was prespecified, found a 31% relative risk reduction ($P$<.05) in the primary outcome in the 17% of patients with TGs greater than 2.3 mmol/L (204 mg/dL) and HDL-C less than 0.9 mmol/L (34 mg/dL), suggesting that fibrates are particularly effective agents in patients with diabetes with low HDL and high TGs. Several additional studies (see **Table 1**) have confirmed these results. There also seems to be a reduction in microvascular and macrovascular diabetic outcomes, such as retinopathy[61] and amputations,[60] for patients with diabetes treated with combination statin-fibrate therapy. A recent meta-analysis reported a 5% reduction in cardiovascular events per a 0.1 mmol/L decrease in TG concentration.[52] Taken together, the evidence suggests that fibrates are effective at lowering TGs and have a marked benefit in patients with diabetes with atherogenic dyslipidemia.

Another pharmacologic agent for treatment of hypertriglyceridemia is niacin. Niacin results in a dose-dependent decrease in plasma TGs (up to 35%) and LDL-C (up to 15%) as well as an increase in HDL-C (up to 25%) via complex mechanisms involving, in part, decreased adipose tissue lipolysis and direct inhibitory effects on TG synthesis.[46,62] The Coronary Drug Project first generated interest in niacin by demonstrating a relative risk reduction of 11% in cardiovascular events and mortality, independent of glycemic control, after 15 years of follow-up.[63,64] It is notable, however, that this was a study comparing niacin against placebo alone; given the overwhelming efficacy of statins, few contemporary patients with dyslipidemia are currently on no background medication. Therefore, in the contemporary population, it is much more relevant to study niacin on a background of statin therapy. The combination of niacin and statin is more effective at lowering TGs, may decrease progression of CAD,[65] and leads to the regression of atherosclerosis, as assessed by carotid intima media thickness.[66] However, the clinical benefit of this combination remains uncertain. The Atherothrombosis Intervention in Metabolic Syndrome with Low HDL-C/High Triglyceride and Impact on Global Health Outcomes (AIM-HIGH) study, which randomized 3414 patients with vascular disease and low HDL on a statin therapy to niacin (Niaspan) versus placebo, attempted to answer this question but was stopped prematurely because of futility. The Data Safety Monitoring Board stopped this trial early because there was no difference in the primary endpoint (composite of coronary death, nonfatal MI, ischemic stroke, ACS requiring hospitalization or revascularization) despite a 25% decrease in TGs and 20% increase in HDL.[67] Therefore, clinical efficacy of lower TGs in this patient population seems limited. Further concerns regarding the impairment of glucose/insulin homeostasis[68] caused by niacin have limited its use despite the resultant improvement in diabetic dyslipidemia.[69] Flushing, another side effect of niacin, is dose dependent and a result of synthesis of prostaglandin D2. The Heart Protection Study2-Treatment of HDL to Reduce the Incidence of Vascular Events (HPS2-THRIVE) is currently investigating a combination of niacin and laropiprant (a prostaglandin antagonist) on a background of statin in 25,000 high-risk patients with metabolic syndrome and diabetes. This new formulation may improve the tolerability of this medication and may identify an important subset of patients who can benefit from the niacin and statin combination. Therefore, although niacin is effective in lowering TG concentrations, its clinical benefit remains to be established.

## POSTPRANDIAL VERSUS FASTING TGS

Because of the surge of TGs following a meal, it has been proposed that fasting TGs may not be the best marker to reflect true risk because they are not reflective of the circulating postprandial lipid levels that the endothelium is exposed to. For this reason, multiple studies have assessed whether postprandial TGs may be superior for predicting coronary outcomes. The Copenhagen city heart study, which enrolled 13,972 patients who were followed in prospective fashion for 31 years, demonstrated that a stepwise increase in nonfasting cholesterol and nonfasting TGs was associated with a stepwise increasing risk of myocardial infarction.[70] Interestingly, the study found that nonfasting TGs were a better predictor of outcomes in women and nonfasting total cholesterol was a better predictor of outcomes in men. Because TG and glucose kinetics are intimately linked, the Homburg cream and sugar study prospectively analyzed whether the degree of TG and glucose tolerance in 500 patients with stable coronary disease correlated with cardiovascular morbidity and mortality at 18 months, in the presence of traditional risk factors.[71] After adjustment in a multivariable model, the study found that neither fasting nor postprandial TGs were predictive of cardiovascular death or cardiovascular hospitalization in the total cohort. However, in the subset of patients with preexisting coronary disease and impaired glucose tolerance, both the fasting and postprandial TGs predicted outcomes. These results highlight the variable role of TGs in predicting risk among heterogeneous patient populations.

## HYPERTRIGLYCERIDEMIA IN SPECIAL POPULATIONS: WOMEN

Neonatal physiology provides early evidence of gender differences in TG concentrations. Female newborns have higher TGs than male newborns,[72] but this difference is rapidly normalized during childhood. Following puberty, TGs decrease in girls and increase in boys.[2] Hormonal variation is seen during menses in lipoprotein and TG levels as well as during pregnancy, although the significance of these changes remains uncertain. Current guidelines recommend screening and risk stratification without adjustment for the phase of the menstrual cycle. Several studies, including the Framingham Heart Study,[73] the Lipid Research Clinics Follow-Up Study,[74] and the Cardiovascular Study in the Elderly,[75] have established that elevated TGs are a predictor of cardiovascular disease and death in women; targets in women are fasting TGs less than 150 mg/dL and non–HDL-C less than 130 mg/dL.[2]

## TGS: HOW MUCH CREDIT DO THEY DESERVE?

The decades-long debate regarding the causal relationship between elevated serum TGs and cardiovascular disease continues to remain unresolved. However, it can be concluded with certainty that, although TGs are a challenging biomarker, elevated concentrations are an important and independent predictor of cardiovascular risk. Decreasing circulating concentrations of this lipid molecule with pharmacologic and nonpharmacologic interventions may translate into improvement in clinical cardiovascular outcomes and mortality. It remains plausible that this protective effect may be amplified in patients with diabetic dyslipidemia (high Tgs and low HDL) and those with metabolic syndrome.

Current recommendations by the American Heart Association/American College of Cardiology and the NCEP ATP III do not include TGs as a primary target for the prevention of CAD. Instead, non–HDL-C (defined as total cholesterol minus HDL cholesterol) is a secondary target,[47] and a recent scientific statement recommends optimal fasting TGs less than 100 mg/dL. However, pending the release of the upcoming ATP IV guidelines, physicians should continue to pay special attention and target lower concentrations of this once under-recognized lipid molecule, which has now emerged as a predictor of adverse clinical outcomes associated with coronary heart disease.

## REFERENCES

1. Hulley SB, Rosenman RH, Bawol RD, et al. Epidemiology as a guide to clinical decisions. The association between triglyceride and coronary heart disease. N Engl J Med 1980;302(25):1383–9.
2. Miller M, Stone NJ, Ballantyne C, et al. Triglycerides and cardiovascular disease: a scientific statement from the American Heart Association. Circulation 2011; 123(20):2292–333.
3. Kearney PM, Blackwell L, Collins R, et al. Efficacy of cholesterol-lowering therapy in 18,686 people with diabetes in 14 randomised trials of statins: a meta-analysis. Lancet 2008;371(9607):117–25.
4. Fruchart JC, Sacks F, Hermans MP, et al. The Residual Risk Reduction Initiative: a call to action to reduce residual vascular risk in patients with dyslipidemia. Am J Cardiol 2008;102(Suppl 10):1K–34K.
5. Brunzell JD, Failor RA. Diagnosis and treatment of dyslipidemia. In: Dale DC, editor. Medicine A, vol. 1. 2006 edition. New York: WebMD; 2006. Available at: http://www.acpmedicine.com/bcdecker/newrxdx/rxdx/dxrx0906.htm. Accessed November 24, 2011.
6. Ford ES, Li C, Zhao G, et al. Hypertriglyceridemia and its pharmacologic treatment among US adults. Arch Intern Med 2009;169(6):572–8.
7. Ginsberg HN. Lipoprotein physiology. Endocrinol Metab Clin North Am 1998; 27(3):503–19.
8. Ginsberg HN. New perspectives on atherogenesis: role of abnormal triglyceride-rich lipoprotein metabolism. Circulation 2002;106(16):2137–42.
9. Watts GF, Karpe F. Triglycerides and atherogenic dyslipidaemia: extending treatment beyond statins in the high-risk cardiovascular patient. Heart 2011;97(5): 350–6.
10. Taskinen MR. Diabetic dyslipidaemia: from basic research to clinical practice. Diabetologia 2003;46(6):733–49.
11. Sarwar N, Sattar N. Triglycerides and coronary heart disease: have recent insights yielded conclusive answers? Curr Opin Lipidol 2009;20(4):275–81.

12. Fox CS, Massaro JM, Hoffmann U, et al. Abdominal visceral and subcutaneous adipose tissue compartments: association with metabolic risk factors in the Framingham Heart Study. Circulation 2007;116(1):39–48.
13. Nicklas BJ, Penninx BW, Ryan AS, et al. Visceral adipose tissue cutoffs associated with metabolic risk factors for coronary heart disease in women. Diabetes Care 2003;26(5):1413–20.
14. Libby P, Bonow R, Mann D, et al, editors. Braunwald's heart disease: a textbook of cardiovascular medicine. 9th edition. Philadelphia: Saunders; 2012.
15. Sarwar N, Sandhu MS, Ricketts SL, et al. Triglyceride-mediated pathways and coronary disease: collaborative analysis of 101 studies. Lancet 2010;375(9726): 1634–9.
16. Friedewald WT, Levy RI, Fredrickson DS. Estimation of the concentration of low-density lipoprotein cholesterol in plasma, without use of the preparative ultracentrifuge. Clin Chem 1972;18(6):499–502.
17. Grundy SM. Hypertriglyceridemia, atherogenic dyslipidemia, and the metabolic syndrome. Am J Cardiol 1998;81(4A):18B–25B.
18. Thorin E. Vascular disease risk in patients with hypertriglyceridemia: endothelial progenitor cells, oxidative stress, accelerated senescence, and impaired vascular repair. Can J Cardiol 2011;27(5):538–40.
19. Yu KC, Cooper AD. Postprandial lipoproteins and atherosclerosis. Front Biosci 2001;6:D332–54.
20. Chait A, Brazg RL, Tribble DL, et al. Susceptibility of small, dense, low-density lipoproteins to oxidative modification in subjects with the atherogenic lipoprotein phenotype, pattern B. Am J Med 1993;94(4):350–6.
21. Kwiterovich PO Jr. Clinical relevance of the biochemical, metabolic, and genetic factors that influence low-density lipoprotein heterogeneity. Am J Cardiol 2002; 90(8A):30i–47i.
22. Greene DJ, Skeggs JW, Morton RE. Elevated triglyceride content diminishes the capacity of high density lipoprotein to deliver cholesteryl esters via the scavenger receptor class B type I (SR-BI). J Biol Chem 2001;276(7):4804–11.
23. Skeggs JW, Morton RE. LDL and HDL enriched in triglyceride promote abnormal cholesterol transport. J Lipid Res 2002;43(8):1264–74.
24. Roncaglioni MC, Santoro L, D'Avanzo B, et al. Role of family history in patients with myocardial infarction. An Italian case-control study. GISSI-EFRIM investigators. Circulation 1992;85(6):2065–72.
25. Genest JJ Jr, Martin-Munley SS, McNamara JR, et al. Familial lipoprotein disorders in patients with premature coronary artery disease. Circulation 1992;85(6): 2025–33.
26. Criqui MH, Heiss G, Cohn R, et al. Plasma triglyceride level and mortality from coronary heart disease. N Engl J Med 1993;328(17):1220–5.
27. Hokanson JE, Austin MA. Plasma triglyceride level is a risk factor for cardiovascular disease independent of high-density lipoprotein cholesterol level: a meta-analysis of population-based prospective studies. J Cardiovasc Risk 1996;3(2): 213–9.
28. Patel A, Barzi F, Jamrozik K, et al. Serum triglycerides as a risk factor for cardiovascular diseases in the Asia-Pacific region. Circulation 2004;110(17): 2678–86.
29. Tirosh A, Rudich A, Shochat T, et al. Changes in triglyceride levels and risk for coronary heart disease in young men. Ann Intern Med 2007;147(6):377–85.
30. Carey VJ, Bishop L, Laranjo N, et al. Contribution of high plasma triglycerides and low high-density lipoprotein cholesterol to residual risk of coronary heart disease

after establishment of low-density lipoprotein cholesterol control. Am J Cardiol 2010;106(6):757–63.

31. Faergeman O, Holme I, Fayyad R, et al. Plasma triglycerides and cardiovascular events in the treating to new targets and incremental decrease in end-points through aggressive lipid lowering trials of statins in patients with coronary artery disease. Am J Cardiol 2009;104(4):459–63.

32. Miller M, Cannon CP, Murphy SA, et al. Impact of triglyceride levels beyond low-density lipoprotein cholesterol after acute coronary syndrome in the PROVE IT-TIMI 22 trial. J Am Coll Cardiol 2008;51(7):724–30.

33. Manninen V, Tenkanen L, Koskinen P, et al. Joint effects of serum triglyceride and LDL cholesterol and HDL cholesterol concentrations on coronary heart disease risk in the Helsinki Heart Study. Implications for treatment. Circulation 1992; 85(1):37–45.

34. Brunzell JD, Deeb SS. Familial lipoprotein lipase deficiency, apo cIII deficiency and hepatic lipase deficiency. In: Scriver CR, Beaudet AL, Sly WD, et al, editors. The metabolic and molecular bases of inherited disease, vol. 3. New York: McGraw-Hill; 2000. p. 2789–816.

35. Brunzell JD, Schrott HG. The interaction of familial and secondary causes of hypertriglyceridemia: role in pancreatitis. Trans Assoc Am Physicians 1973;86:245–54.

36. Birjmohun RS, Hutten BA, Kastelein JJ, et al. Efficacy and safety of high-density lipoprotein cholesterol-increasing compounds: a meta-analysis of randomized controlled trials. J Am Coll Cardiol 2005;45(2):185–97.

37. Purnell JQ, Kahn SE, Albers JJ, et al. Effect of weight loss with reduction of intra-abdominal fat on lipid metabolism in older men. J Clin Endocrinol Metab 2000; 85(3):977–82.

38. Knowler WC, Barrett-Connor E, Fowler SE, et al. Reduction in the incidence of type 2 diabetes with lifestyle intervention or metformin. N Engl J Med 2002; 346(6):393–403.

39. Lichtenstein AH, Appel LJ, Brands M, et al. Summary of American Heart Association diet and lifestyle recommendations revision 2006. Arterioscler Thromb Vasc Biol 2006;26(10):2186–91.

40. Lichtenstein AH, Appel LJ, Brands M, et al. Diet and lifestyle recommendations revision 2006: a scientific statement from the American Heart Association Nutrition Committee. Circulation 2006;114(1):82–96.

41. Brunzell JD. Clinical practice. Hypertriglyceridemia. N Engl J Med 2007;357(10): 1009–17.

42. Leon AS, Sanchez OA. Response of blood lipids to exercise training alone or combined with dietary intervention. Med Sci Sports Exerc 2001;33(Suppl 6): S502–15 [discussion: S528–9].

43. Ross R, Dagnone D, Jones PJ, et al. Reduction in obesity and related comorbid conditions after diet-induced weight loss or exercise-induced weight loss in men. A randomized, controlled trial. Ann Intern Med 2000;133(2):92–103.

44. Havel PJ. Dietary fructose: implications for dysregulation of energy homeostasis and lipid/carbohydrate metabolism. Nutr Rev 2005;63(5):133–57.

45. Phillips NR, Havel RJ, Kane JP. Levels and interrelationships of serum and lipoprotein cholesterol and triglycerides. Association with adiposity and the consumption of ethanol, tobacco, and beverages containing caffeine. Arteriosclerosis 1981;1(1):13–24.

46. Chan DC, Watts GF. Dyslipidaemia in the metabolic syndrome and type 2 diabetes: pathogenesis, priorities, pharmacotherapies. Expert Opin Pharmacother 2011;12(1):13–30.

47. Grundy SM, Cleeman JI, Merz CN, et al. Implications of recent clinical trials for the National Cholesterol Education Program Adult Treatment Panel III guidelines. Circulation 2004;110(2):227–39.
48. Gibson CM, Pride YB, Hochberg CP, et al. Effect of intensive statin therapy on clinical outcomes among patients undergoing percutaneous coronary intervention for acute coronary syndrome. PCI-PROVE IT: a PROVE IT-TIMI 22 (Pravastatin or Atorvastatin Evaluation and Infection Therapy-Thrombolysis In Myocardial Infarction 22) substudy. J Am Coll Cardiol 2009;54(24):2290–5.
49. Shepherd J, Barter P, Carmena R, et al. Effect of lowering LDL cholesterol substantially below currently recommended levels in patients with coronary heart disease and diabetes: the Treating to New Targets (TNT) study. Diabetes Care 2006;29(6): 1220–6.
50. Colhoun HM, Betteridge DJ, Durrington PN, et al. Primary prevention of cardiovascular disease with atorvastatin in type 2 diabetes in the Collaborative Atorvastatin Diabetes Study (CARDS): multicentre randomised placebo-controlled trial. Lancet 2004;364(9435):685–96.
51. Ginsberg HN, Elam MB, Lovato LC, et al. Effects of combination lipid therapy in type 2 diabetes mellitus. N Engl J Med 2010;362(17):1563–74.
52. Jun M, Foote C, Lv J, et al. Effects of fibrates on cardiovascular outcomes: a systematic review and meta-analysis. Lancet 2010;375(9729):1875–84.
53. Keech A, Simes RJ, Barter P, et al. Effects of long-term fenofibrate therapy on cardiovascular events in 9795 people with type 2 diabetes mellitus (the FIELD study): randomised controlled trial. Lancet 2005;366(9500):1849–61.
54. Staels B, Dallongeville J, Auwerx J, et al. Mechanism of action of fibrates on lipid and lipoprotein metabolism. Circulation 1998;98(19):2088–93.
55. Marx N, Duez H, Fruchart JC, et al. Peroxisome proliferator-activated receptors and atherogenesis: regulators of gene expression in vascular cells. Circ Res 2004;94(9):1168–78.
56. Goldfine AB, Kaul S, Hiatt WR. Fibrates in the treatment of dyslipidemias–time for a reassessment. N Engl J Med 2011;365(6):481–4.
57. Frick MH, Elo O, Haapa K, et al. Helsinki Heart Study: primary-prevention trial with gemfibrozil in middle-aged men with dyslipidemia. Safety of treatment, changes in risk factors, and incidence of coronary heart disease. N Engl J Med 1987; 317(20):1237–45.
58. Rubins HB, Robins SJ, Collins D, et al. Gemfibrozil for the secondary prevention of coronary heart disease in men with low levels of high-density lipoprotein cholesterol. Veterans Affairs High-Density Lipoprotein Cholesterol Intervention Trial Study Group. N Engl J Med 1999;341(6):410–8.
59. BIP Study Group. Secondary prevention by raising HDL cholesterol and reducing triglycerides in patients with coronary artery disease: the Bezafibrate Infarction Prevention (BIP) study. Circulation 2000;102(1):21–7.
60. Scott R, O'Brien R, Fulcher G, et al. Effects of fenofibrate treatment on cardiovascular disease risk in 9,795 individuals with type 2 diabetes and various components of the metabolic syndrome: the Fenofibrate Intervention and Event Lowering in Diabetes (FIELD) study. Diabetes Care 2009;32(3):493–8.
61. Ambrosius WT, Danis RP, Goff DC Jr, et al. Lack of association between thiazolidinediones and macular edema in type 2 diabetes: the ACCORD eye substudy. Arch Ophthalmol 2010;128(3):312–8.
62. Chapman MJ, Redfern JS, McGovern ME, et al. Niacin and fibrates in atherogenic dyslipidemia: pharmacotherapy to reduce cardiovascular risk. Pharmacol Ther 2010;126(3):314–45.

63. Canner PL, Berge KG, Wenger NK, et al. Fifteen year mortality in Coronary Drug Project patients: long-term benefit with niacin. J Am Coll Cardiol 1986;8(6):1245–55.

64. Canner PL, Furberg CD, Terrin ML, et al. Benefits of niacin by glycemic status in patients with healed myocardial infarction (from the Coronary Drug Project). Am J Cardiol 2005;95(2):254–7.

65. Brown BG, Zhao XQ, Chait A, et al. Simvastatin and niacin, antioxidant vitamins, or the combination for the prevention of coronary disease. N Engl J Med 2001; 345(22):1583–92.

66. Taylor AJ, Sullenberger LE, Lee HJ, et al. Arterial Biology for the Investigation of the Treatment Effects of Reducing Cholesterol (ARBITER) 2: a double-blind, placebo-controlled study of extended-release niacin on atherosclerosis progression in secondary prevention patients treated with statins. Circulation 2004; 110(23):3512–7.

67. The AIM-HIGH investigators. The role of niacin in raising high-density lipoprotein cholesterol to reduce cardiovascular events in patients with atherosclerotic cardiovascular disease and optimally treated low-density lipoprotein cholesterol Rationale and study design. The Atherothrombosis Intervention in Metabolic syndrome with low HDL/high triglycerides: impact on Global Health outcomes (AIM-HIGH). Am Heart J 2011;161(3):471–7, e472.

68. Guyton JR, Bays HE. Safety considerations with niacin therapy. Am J Cardiol 2007;99(6A):22C–31C.

69. Grundy SM, Vega GL, McGovern ME, et al. Efficacy, safety, and tolerability of once-daily niacin for the treatment of dyslipidemia associated with type 2 diabetes: results of the assessment of diabetes control and evaluation of the efficacy of Niaspan trial. Arch Intern Med 2002;162(14):1568–76.

70. Langsted A, Freiberg JJ, Tybjaerg-Hansen A, et al. Nonfasting cholesterol and triglycerides and association with risk of myocardial infarction and total mortality: the Copenhagen City Heart Study with 31 years of follow-up. J Intern Med 2011; 270(1):65–75.

71. Laufs U. The correlation of triglyceride and glucose tolerance with cardiovascular outcomes in patients with stable coronary artery disease: the Homburg Cream and Sugar study (HCS). Paper presented at: European Society of Cardiology Congress 2011. HOTLINE sessions at ESC, Paris (France), August 28, 2011.

72. Bansal N, Cruickshank JK, McElduff P, et al. Cord blood lipoproteins and prenatal influences. Curr Opin Lipidol 2005;16(4):400–8.

73. Castelli WP. The triglyceride issue: a view from Framingham. Am Heart J 1986; 112(2):432–7.

74. Bass KM, Newschaffer CJ, Klag MJ, et al. Plasma lipoprotein levels as predictors of cardiovascular death in women. Arch Intern Med 1993;153(19):2209–16.

75. Mazza A, Tikhonoff V, Schiavon L, et al. Triglycerides + high-density-lipoprotein-cholesterol dyslipidaemia, a coronary risk factor in elderly women: the CArdiovascular STudy in the ELderly. Intern Med J 2005;35(10):604–10.

76. Tuomilehto J, Lindstrom J, Eriksson JG, et al. Prevention of type 2 diabetes mellitus by changes in lifestyle among subjects with impaired glucose tolerance. N Engl J Med 2001;344(18):1343–50.

77. Van Gaal LF, Mertens IL, Ballaux D. What is the relationship between risk factor reduction and degree of weight loss? Eur Heart J Suppl 2005;7(Suppl):L21–6.

78. Anderson JW, Konz EC. Obesity and disease management: effects of weight loss on comorbid conditions. Obesity 2001;9(11S):326S–34S.

79. Dattilo A, Kris-Etherton P. Effects of weight reduction on blood lipids and lipoproteins: a meta- analysis. Am J Clin Nutr 1992;56(2):320–8.

80. Erkelens DW, Brunzell JD. Effect of controlled alcohol feeding on triglycerides in patients with outpatient 'alcohol hypertriglyceridemia'. J Hum Nutr 1980;34(5):370–5.
81. Rimm EB, Williams P, Fosher K, et al. Moderate alcohol intake and lower risk of coronary heart disease: meta-analysis of effects on lipids and haemostatic factors. BMJ 1999;319(7224):1523–8.
82. Cannon CP, Braunwald E, McCabe CH, et al. Intensive versus moderate lipid lowering with statins after acute coronary syndromes. N Engl J Med 2004; 350(15):1495–504.
83. Baigent C, Blackwell L, Emberson J, et al. Efficacy and safety of more intensive lowering of LDL cholesterol: a meta-analysis of data from 170,000 participants in 26 randomised trials. Lancet 2010;376(9753):1670–81.
84. Clofibrate and niacin in coronary heart disease. JAMA 1975;231(4):360–81.
85. Goldberg RB, Guyton JR, Mazzone T, et al. Ezetimibe/simvastatin vs atorvastatin in patients with type 2 diabetes mellitus and hypercholesterolemia: the VYTAL study. Mayo Clin Proc 2006;81(12):1579–88.
86. Dietary supplementation with n-3 polyunsaturated fatty acids and vitamin E after myocardial infarction: results of the GISSI-Prevenzione trial. Gruppo Italiano per lo Studio della Sopravvivenza nell'Infarto miocardico. Lancet 1999;354(9177): 447–55.
87. Yokoyama M, Origasa H, Matsuzaki M, et al. Effects of eicosapentaenoic acid on major coronary events in hypercholesterolaemic patients (JELIS): a randomised open-label, blinded endpoint analysis. Lancet 2007;369(9567):1090–8.
88. Balk E, Chung M, Lichtenstein A, et al. Effects of omega-3 fatty acids on cardiovascular risk factors and intermediate markers of cardiovascular disease. Evid Rep Technol Assess (Summ) 2004;93:1–6.
89. Harris WS. n-3 fatty acids and serum lipoproteins: human studies. Am J Clin Nutr 1997;65(Suppl 5):1645S–54S.

# Atherosclerosis in Chronic Kidney Disease: Lessons Learned from Glycation in Diabetes

Dilbahar S. Mohar, MD[a,b,]*, Ailin Barseghian, MD[a,b,]*,
Nezam Haider, PhD[a,b], Michael Domanski, MD[a,b],
Jagat Narula, MD, PhD[a,b]

**KEYWORDS**

- Glycation • Carbamylation • Advanced glycated end products
- Atherosclerosis • Cardiovascular disease

Certain disease processes may modify proteins in the vessel wall in a way that contributes to the development and progression of atherosclerosis. In diabetes, glycation is a nonenzymatic posttranslational modification resulting from the bonding of a sugar molecule with a protein or lipid followed by oxidation, resulting in the development of advanced glycation end products (AGE). Glycation of extracellular matrix (ECM) proteins and low-density lipoprotein (LDL) with subsequent deposition in the vessel wall could contribute to inflammatory response and atheroma formation.[1,2] Because vascular pathology in chronic kidney disease (CKD) is not clearly understood and elevated urea may be as reactive, it is logical to extrapolate that the process of carbamylation may result in modification of vessel wall proteins similar to glycation, and predispose to atherosclerosis.

## GLYCATION AND ATHEROSCLEROSIS IN DIABETES

In patients with diabetes, free amino groups located at either the N-terminal and/or lysl-hydroxylysyl side chains undergo nonenzymatic glycation followed by oxidation of these ketoamine products, leading to formation of AGE (**Fig. 1**).[3,4] Vessel wall

D.M. and A.B. contributed equally to this article.
[a] Division of Cardiology, University of California-Irvine School of Medicine, 333 City Boulevard West, Suite 400, Orange, CA 92868-3298, USA
[b] Mount Sinai School of Medicine, 1 Gustave L. Levy Place, Box 1030, New York, NY 10029-6574, USA
* Corresponding author. Division of Cardiology, University of California-Irvine School of Medicine, 333 City Boulevard West, Suite 400, Orange, CA 92868-3298.
*E-mail addresses:* dmohar@uci.edu; barsegha@uci.edu

Med Clin N Am 96 (2012) 57–65
doi:10.1016/j.mcna.2011.11.005
0025-7125/12/$ – see front matter © 2012 Elsevier Inc. All rights reserved.

medical.theclinics.com

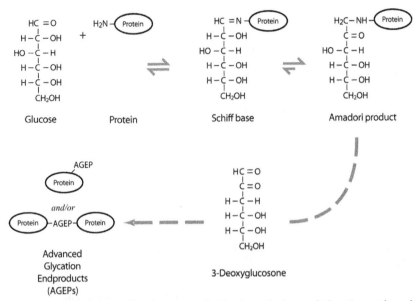

**Fig. 1.** Glycation reaction and end products. Production of advanced glycation end products (AGE) via the glycation of proteins involves: (1) formation of a Schiff base, (2) rearrangement to an Amadori product, and (3) irreversible oxidation of the Amadori product to the formation of a reactive electrophilic species able to react with proteins to form AGE. (*From* Ahmad MS, Ahmed N. Antiglycation properties of aged garlic extract: possible role in prevention of diabetic complications. J Nutr 2006;136:797; with permission.)

AGE deposition[1,5,6] is progressive, and causes irreversible cross-linking and polymerization of extracellular matrix proteins such as collagen, resulting in the loss of elasticity and increased stiffness of the vasculature.[7–10] Alterations in extracellular substrate may result in endothelial dysfunction and may perpetuate the process of lipid permeation,[11,12] monocyte recruitment,[13] and proliferation of smooth muscle cells (SMC) (**Table 1**).[3,14] Strict control of blood glucose in patients with type 2 diabetes mellitus (DM)[15–17] have not demonstrated incremental value for prevention of macrovascular complications at the time of the conclusion of studies such as ACCORD, ADVANCE, and VADT. However, posttrial monitoring of the UKPDS study patients at 10 years demonstrated risk reduction for all macrovascular outcomes, including myocardial infarction and death from any cause.[18] It is of interest to determine whether the legacy effect is the result of an underlying process that affected the coronary artery disease (CAD)-naïve patient population of the UKPDS trial that was not modifiable in the patient population with preexisting CAD in the other studies. Thus, a possible explanation may be that protein modifications in diabetics result in irreversible damage to the arterial wall and provide a basis for susceptibility to CAD. The stability of the proteins is highly dependent on the presence of the N-terminal amino acid (N-end rule), and is enhanced with glycation. Unlike glycated circulating proteins, which possess only a limited half-life of several months, glycated extracellular matrix (ECM) proteins may demonstrate greater resistance to degradation and prolonged half-lives. Therefore, glycation of ECM proteins may induce an irreversible modification to the arterial wall and create an ideal environment for progressive long-term atherosclerotic disease, and hence a legacy effect.[18]

**Table 1**
**Posttranslational modification of proteins in cardiovascular disease diabetes and CKD**

| Substrate | Effect |
|---|---|
| Glycation | |
| LDL | Increased LDL accumulation as enhanced proteoglycan binding leads to increased lipid deposition and decreased clearance of LDL |
| Collagen | Increases release of growth modulators, resulting in thickening of basement membrane. Increased resistance and decreased elasticity of vessel wall |
| Fibrin | Increased thickening of basement membrane. Proliferation of vascular smooth muscle cells |
| Proteoglycans, fibronectin | Altered ECM organization as affinity of collagen to basement membrane decreased |
| Elastin, laminin | Increased stiffness and calcium deposition, imparts decreased compliance of vessel wall |
| Carbamylation | |
| LDL | Increased endothelial cell apoptosis, diminished LDL-receptor recognition, increased foam-cell formation, and proliferation of smooth muscle cells |
| Collagen | Creates disorganized fibrillar tissue in ECM, inhibits incorporation of newly synthesized collagen, increases release of matrix metalloproteinases, increases cell proinflammatory markers and adhesion molecules such as ICAM-1 and VCAM-1 |
| Fibrin | Increases basement membrane thickening |
| Proteoglycans, fibronectin | Alters ECM organization as affinity of collagen to basement membrane decreased |

*Abbreviations:* ECM, extracellular matrix; ICAM, intracellular adhesion molecule; LDL, low-density lipoprotein; VCAM, vascular cell adhesion molecule.

ECM proteins, such as collagen, elastin, fibronectin, laminin, and proteoglycans, are preferential targets for posttranslational modifications because they possess longer half-lives and are thus exposed to a greater burden of oxidative stress. One of the more abundant proteins of the ECM, collagen is a prime target for long-term glycation. Type I collagen has a low biological turnover rate and possesses numerous lysine and hydroxylysine residues. Thickening of the basement membrane, as seen commonly in diabetic vasculature, may be the consequence of membrane binding of growth modulators promoted by collagen glycation.[19–21] Furthermore, glycation of type IV collagen alters the scaffolding properties and restricts endothelial attachment to the basement membrane.[22] In comprehensive terms, the structural dynamics of diabetic vessels are compromised as glycosylated collagen imparts relative resistance to degradation and decreased elasticity to the vessel wall.

Whereas collagen ultimately determines tensile strength in tissue, elastin is mainly responsible for compliance of the vessel wall. Possessing the lowest turnover rate of all ECM proteins, elastin is a preferential target for glycation[10] that contributes to increased stiffness.[23,24] Laminins are basal lamina proteins whose glycation hinders the endothelial cell adhesion and spread.[22] On the other hand, proteoglycans and fibronectin are responsible for matrix self-assembly and are associated with the structure of the basement membrane. Glycation of these proteins results in altered matrix

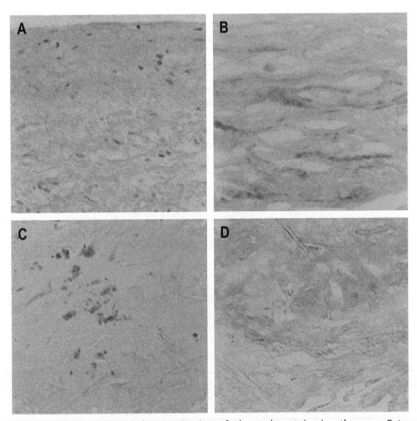

**Fig. 2.** Immunohistochemical characterization of glycated proteins in atheroma. Extracellular AGE deposition is depicted using immunohistochemical staining of human atherosclerotic lesions with an AGE antibody. The diffusely thickened intimal area reveals positive AGE-antibody staining (*A*) and extracellular AGE deposits in hyalinized collagen fibers (*B*). On the other hand, the central atheroma depicts fine granular (*C*) and diffuse (*D*) AGE deposition. (*From* Kume M, Takeya T, Mori N, et al. Immunohistochemical and ultrastructural detection of advanced glycation end products in atherosclerotic lesions of human aorta with a novel specific monoclonal antibody. Am J Pathol 1995;147:659; with permission.)

organization and a decreased affinity to collagen in the basement membrane.[25] In addition, glycosylated fibrin accumulates in the basement membrane and contributes to thickening. Accumulation of fibrin in the arterial wall also enhances the proliferation of vascular SMC.[26] Similarly, prelesional low-density lipoprotein (LDL) retention in the ECM has been associated with the initial pathogenesis of atherosclerosis.[27] Proteoglycans in the arterial wall are major components of lipid binding.[28] Glycation of LDL enhances proteoglycan binding of LDL and increases lipid deposition.[27] Glycation further potentiates accumulation of vascular wall LDL as degradation and clearance of the modified, glycated LDL is decreased in comparison with native LDL (**Fig. 2**).[29–32]

## CARBAMYLATION OF VASCULAR PROTEINS AS A CONTRIBUTOR TO ATHEROSCLEROSIS

Historically carbamylation has been reported with the treatment of sickle cell disease,[33–35] chronicity of uremia,[36] and its interference in the accurate measurement of hemoglobin $A_{1c}$ in diabetic patients.[37] Carbamylation causes changes in protein conformation, leading to altered protein-protein or protein-cell interactions.[38] Like glycation, carbamylation is a posttranslational protein modification that is associated with AGE formation. Furthermore, systemic carbamylated proteins have been strongly associated with prevalence of cardiovascular disease, risk of future major adverse cardiac events, and degree of atherosclerotic inflammatory changes relative to normal vascular tissue.[39]

The primary carbamylation process involves an unprotonated cyanate undergoing reaction with the N-terminal amino acid or lysine residue of an individual protein.[40,41] The process results in the production of a highly reactive oxidized homocitrulline molecule anchored within long-lived vessel protein. The resulting carbamylated proteins are increasingly resistant to enzymatic digestion, and their life span is extended.[39] Further, production of the cyanate-group reactant required for carbamylation evolves by either of two reactions: the extensively studied uremia-mediated process or the more novel myeloperoxidase (MPO)-mediated reaction (**Fig. 3**).[39] Uremia-mediated protein carbamylation is dependent on both the duration and concentration of urea exposure.[36,42–44] On the other hand, MPO in inflammatory states may catalyze the reaction of the substrates thiocyanate and hydrogen peroxide to produce cyanate, the principal molecule of protein carbamylation.[39] MPO is highly expressed in neutrophils, monocytes, and macrophages found in atheromas (**Fig. 4**).[45,46] Regardless of

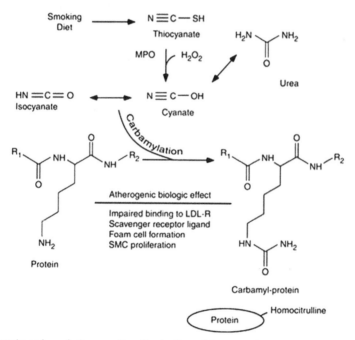

**Fig. 3.** Protein carbamylation reaction. Production of the cyanate group reactant required for vessel-wall protein carbamylation is facilitated by either the uremia-mediated or a myeloperoxidase (MPO)-mediated reaction. Uremia-mediated cyanate production is enhanced, as an equilibrium between urea and cyanate exists in renal disease. MPO, a prominent enzyme found in inflammatory states, catalyzes the reaction between thiocyanate (SCN) and hydrogen peroxide (H₂O₂) to produce cyanate (OCN). LDL-R, low-density lipoprotein receptor; SMC, smooth muscle cells. (*From* Wang Z, Nicholls SJ, Rodriguez ER, et al. Protein carbamylation links inflammation, smoking, uremia and atherogenesis. Nat Med 2007;13:1177; with permission.)

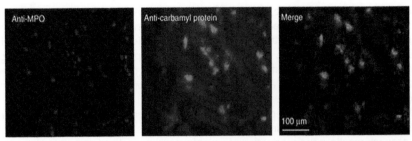

**Fig. 4.** Immunofluorescence characterization for carbamylated proteins. Human carotid atherosclerotic plaque is immunostained with monoclonal antibodies to MPO (*left*) or carbamyl proteins (*center*). The merged image (*right*) depicts their colocalization. Nuclei were stained with DAPI (4′, 6-diamidino-2-phenylindole) (*blue*). (*From* Wang Z, Nicholls SJ, Rodriguez ER, et al. Protein carbamylation links inflammation, smoking, uremia and atherogenesis. Nat Med 2007;13:1178; with permission.)

the mode of cyanate production, protein carbamylation causes endothelial dysfunction and potentiates susceptibility to atherosclerosis (see **Table 1**).[47]

Carbamylation of collagen has been shown to alter the structure and function of the ECM. It creates a disorganized fibrillar tissue structure by interfering with the growth of fibrils, and impairs the incorporation of the newly synthesized collagen molecules.[38] Carbamylated type I collagen elicits adhesion and activation of monocytes through interactions with integrins, and potentiates cell adhesion and proinflammatory markers.[48] In addition, carbamylated type I collagen exaggerates the release of matrix metalloproteinases,[49] which may contribute to the degradation of the basement membrane, compromise the endothelial barrier,[50] and potentiate vascular remodeling.[49]

Relative to traditional LDL, carbamylated LDL (cLDL) markedly increases the risk of atherosclerotic disease. cLDL has been reported to possess numerous proatherogenic properties, including increased endothelial apoptosis and diminished LDL-receptor recognition, leading to decreased clearance and retention of LDL in the vascular wall.[32,51] Furthermore, cLDL has been noted to induce monocyte adhesion,[52] increase macrophage accumulation by intensifying receptor recognition of LDL,[39] augment foam cell formation,[39] and promote proliferation of vascular smooth cells.[47,53,54]

## SUMMARY

The accelerated rate of atherogenesis in the diabetic population may be facilitated by posttranslational protein modifications, such as glycation and carbamylation, and may provide a clue as to the inciting events that result in atherosclerosis. Furthermore, it has been suggested that cross-links formed by glycated moieties can be reversed by cross-link inhibitors such as aminoguanidines.[55,56] These findings suggest that prevention of the irreversible glycated and carbamylated products may become plausible, and may hold promise for the prevention of atherosclerosis.

## REFERENCES

1. Nakamura Y, Horii Y, Nishino T, et al. Immunohistochemical localization of advanced glycosylation end products in coronary atheroma and cardiac tissue in diabetes mellitus. Am J Pathol 1993;143(6):1649–56.

2. Sakata N, Imanaga Y, Meng J, et al. Increased advanced glycation end products in atherosclerotic lesions of patients with end-stage renal disease. Atherosclerosis 1999;142(1):67–77.
3. Cerami A, Vlassara H, Brownlee M. Role of nonenzymatic glycosylation in atherogenesis. J Cell Biochem 1986;30(2):111–20.
4. Gillery P, Monboisse JC, Maquart FX, et al. Aging mechanisms of proteins [abstract only]. Diabetes Metab 1991;17(1):1–16.
5. Vogt BW, Schleicher ED, Wieland OH. ε-Amino-lysine-bound glucose in human tissues obtained at autopsy increase in diabetes mellitus. Diabetes 1982;31: 1123–7.
6. Palinski W, Koschinsky T, Butler SW, et al. Immunological evidence for the presence of advanced glycosylation end products in atherosclerotic lesions of euglycemic rabbits. Arterioscler Thromb Vasc Biol 1995;15:571–82.
7. Eble AS, Thorpe SR, Baynes JW. Nonenzymatic glucosylation and glucose-dependent cross-linking of protein. J Biol Chem 1983;258(15):9406–12.
8. Brownlee M, Cerami A, Vlassara H. Advanced products of nonenzymatic glycosylation and the pathogenesis of diabetic vascular disease. Diabetes Metab Rev 1988;4(5):437–51.
9. Aronson D. Cross-linking of glycated collagen in the pathogenesis of arterial and myocardial stiffening of aging and diabetes. J Hypertens 2003;21(1): 3–12.
10. Paul RG, Bailey AJ. Glycation of collagen: the basis of its central role in the late complications of ageing and diabetes. Int J Biochem Cell Biol 1996;28(12): 1297–310.
11. Vlassara H. Advanced glycation end-products and atherosclerosis. Ann Med 1996;28(5):419–26.
12. Meng J, Sakata N, Takebayashi S, et al. Glycoxidation in aortic collagen from STZ-induced diabetic rats and its relevance to vascular damage. Atherosclerosis 1998;136(2):355–65.
13. Kirstein M, Brett J, Radoff S, et al. Advanced protein glycosylation induces trans-endothelial human monocyte chemotaxis and secretion of platelet-derived growth factor: role in vascular disease of diabetes and aging. Proc Natl Acad Sci U S A 1990;87(22):9010–4.
14. Sakata N, Meng J, Takebayashi S. Effects of advanced glycation end products on the proliferation and fibronectin production of smooth muscle cells. J Atheroscler Thromb 2000;7(3):169–76.
15. Gerstein HC, Miller ME, Byington RP, et al. Action to Control Cardiovascular Risk in Diabetes Study Group (ACCORD), Effects of intensive glucose lowering in type 2 diabetes. N Engl J Med 2008;358(24):2545–59.
16. Patel A, MacMahon S, Chalmers J, et al. ADVANCE Collaborative Group, Intensive blood glucose control and vascular outcomes in patients with type 2 diabetes. N Engl J Med 2008;385(24):2560–72.
17. Duckworth W, Abraira C, Moritz T, et al. Glucose control and vascular complications in veterans with type 2 diabetes (VADT). N Engl J Med 2009;360(2): 129–39.
18. Holman RR, Paul SK, Bethel MA, et al. 10-Year follow-up of intensive glucose control in type 2 diabetes. N Engl J Med 2008;359(15):1577–89.
19. Lubec G, Pollak A. Reduced susceptibility of nonenzymatically glucosylated glomerular basement membrane to proteases: is thickening of diabetic glomerular basement membranes due to reduced proteolytic degradation? Ren Physiol 1980;3(1–6):4–8.

20. Brownlee M, Pongor S, Cerami A. Covalent attachment of soluble proteins by nonenzymatically glycosylated collagen. Role in the in situ formation of immune complexes. J Exp Med 1983;158(5):1739–44.

21. Tsilibary EC. Microvascular basement membranes in diabetes mellitus. J Pathol 2003;200(4):537–46.

22. Haitoglou CS, Tsilibary EC, Brownlee M, et al. Altered cellular interactions between endothelial cells and nonenzymatically glucosylated laminin/type IV collagen. J Biol Chem 1992;267(18):12404–7.

23. Tomizawa H, Yamazaki M, Kunika K, et al. Association of elastin glycation and calcium deposit in diabetic rat aorta. Diabetes Res Clin Pract 1993;19(1):1–8.

24. Winlove CP, Parker KH, Avery NC, et al. Interactions of elastin and aorta with sugars in vitro and their effects on biochemical and physical properties. Diabetologia 1996;39(10):1131–9.

25. Tarsio JF, Reger LA, Furcht LT. Decreased interaction of fibronectin, type IV collagen, and heparin due to nonenzymatic glycation. Implications for diabetes mellitus. Biochemistry 1987;26:1014–20.

26. Ishida T, Tanaka K. Effects of fibrin and fibrinogen-degradation products on the growth of rabbit aortic smooth muscle cells in culture. Atherosclerosis 1982;44(2):161–74.

27. Edwards IJ, Wagner JD, Litwak KN, et al. Glycation of plasma low density lipoproteins increases interaction with arterial proteoglycans. Diabetes Res Clin Pract 1999;46:9–18.

28. Little PJ, Ballinger ML, Osman N. Vascular wall proteoglycan synthesis and structure as a target for the prevention of atherosclerosis. Vasc Health Risk Manag 2007;3(1):117–24.

29. Sasaki J, Cottam GL. Glycosylatin of LDL decreases its ability to interact with high-affinity receptors of human fibroblasts in vitro and decreases its clearance from rabbit plasma in vivo. Biochim Biophys Acta 1982;713:199–207.

30. Witztum JL, Mahoney EM, Branks MJ, et al. Nonenzymatic glucosylation of low-density lipoprotein alters its biologic activity. Diabetes 1982;31(4 Pt 1):283–91.

31. Steinbrecher UP, Witztum JL. Glucosylation of low-density lipoproteins to an extent comparable to that seen in diabetes slows their catabolism. Diabetes 1984;33:130–4.

32. Hörkkö S, Huttunen K, Antero Kesaniemi Y. Decreased clearance of low-density lipoprotein in uremic patients under dialysis treatment. Kidney Int 1995;47:1732–40.

33. Gillette PN, Manning JM, Cerami A. Increased survival of sickle-cell erythrocytes after treatment in vitro with sodium cyanate. Proc Natl Acad Sci U S A 1971;68(11):2791–3.

34. Cerami A. Cyanate as an inhibitor of red-cell sickling. N Engl J Med 1972;287:807–12.

35. Deiderich DA, Trueworthy RC, Gill P, et al. Hematologic and clinical responses in patients with sickle cell anemia after chronic extracorporeal red cell carbamylation. J Clin Invest 1976;58(3):642–53.

36. Flückiger R, Harmon W, Meier W, et al. Hemoglobin carbamylation in uremia. N Engl J Med 1981;304:823–7.

37. Chachou A, Randoux C, Millart H, et al. Influence of in vivo hemoglobin carbamylation on HbA1c measurements by various methods. Clin Chem Lab Med 2000;38:321–6.

38. Jaisson S, Lorimier S, Ricard-Blum S, et al. Impact of carbamylation on type I collagen conformational structure and its ability to activate human polymorphonuclear neutrophils. Chem Biol 2006;13(2):149–59.

39. Wang Z, Nicholls SJ, Rodriguez ER, et al. Protein carbamylation links inflammation, smoking, uremia and atherogenesis. Nat Med 2007;13:1176–84.
40. Stark GR. Reactions of cyanate with functional groups of proteins. 3. Reactions with amino and carboxyl groups. Biochemistry 1965;4:1030–6.
41. Kraus LM, Kraus AP Jr. Carbamoylation of amino acids and proteins in uremia. Kidney Int Suppl 2001;78:S102–7.
42. Han JS, Kim YS, Chin HI, et al. Temporal changes and reversibility of carbamylated hemoglobin in renal failure. Am J Kidney Dis 1997;30:36–40.
43. Kwan JT, Carr EC, Barron JL, et al. Carbamylated haemoglobin—a retrospective index of time-averaged urea concentration. Nephrol Dial Transplant 1993;8: 565–7.
44. Davenport A, Jones S, Goel S, et al. Carbamylated hemoglobin: a potential marker for the adequacy of hemodialysis therapy in end-stage renal failure. Kidney Int 1996;50:1344–51.
45. Zhang R, Brennan ML, Fu X, et al. Association between myeloperoxidase levels and risk of coronary artery disease. JAMA 2001;286(17):2136–42.
46. Rudolph TK, Wipper S, Reiter B, et al. Myeloperoxidase deficiency preserves vasomotor function in humans. Eur Heart J 2011;1–10.
47. Ok E, Basnakian AG, Apostolov EO, et al. Carbamylated low-density lipoprotein induces death of endothelial cells: a link to atherosclerosis in patients with kidney disease. Kidney Int 2005;68:173–8.
48. Garnotel R, Rittié L, Poitevin S, et al. Human blood monocytes interact with type I collagen through alpha x beta 2 integrin (CD11c-CD18, gp150-95). J Immunol 2000;164(11):5928–34.
49. Garnotel R, Sabbah N, Jaisson S, et al. Enhanced activation of and increased production of matrix metalloproteinase-9 by human blood monocytes upon adhering to carbamylated collagen. FEBS Lett 2004;563(1–3):13–6.
50. Rosenberg GA, Estrada EY, Dencoff JE. Matrix metalloproteinases and TIMPs are associated with blood-brain barrier opening after reperfusion in rat brain. Stroke 1998;29(10):2189–95.
51. Hörkkö S, Huttunen K, Kervinen K, et al. Decreased clearance of uraemic and mildly carbamylated low-density lipoprotein. Eur J Clin Invest 1994;24:105–13.
52. Apostolov EO, Shah SV, Ok E, et al. Carbamylated low density lipoprotein induces monocyte adhesion to endothelial cells through intercellular adhesion molecule 1 and vascular cell adhesion molecule 1. Arterioscler Thromb Vasc Biol 2007;27:826–32.
53. Asci G, Basci A, Shah SV, et al. Carbamylated low-density lipoprotein induces proliferation and increases adhesion molecule expression of human coronary artery smooth muscle cells. Nephrology 2008;13(6):480–6.
54. Shah SV, Apostolov EO, Ok E, et al. Novel mechanisms in accelerated atherosclerosis in kidney disease. J Ren Nutr 2008;18(1):65–9.
55. Brownlee M, Vlassara H, Kooney T, et al. Aminoguanidine prevents diabetes-induced arterial wall protein cross-linking. Science 1986;232:1629–32.
56. Charonis AS, Reger LA, Dege JE, et al. Laminin alterations after in vitro nonenzymatic glycosylation. Diabetes 1990;39(7):807–14.

# "My Parents Died of Myocardial Infarction: Is that My Destiny?"

Nupoor Narula, BS[a], Claudio Rapezzi, MD, FESC[b],
Luigi Tavazzi, MD[c], Eloisa Arbustini, MD, PhD[a],*

**KEYWORDS**

• Myocardial infarction • Genetics • Family history • Risk factors

Myocardial infarction (MI) is a multifactorial and multistep event that occurs when an acute thrombus occludes a vulnerable coronary atherosclerotic artery.[1] MI depends on the complex interplay between genetic and environmental factors, including unpredictable and unpreventable exogenous triggers.[2]

A positive family history for MI constitutes one of the most significant independent risk factors for MI. Hardly a day goes by without hearing questions from patients informed by the media about discoveries in the genetics of MI, concerned that some of their closest relatives died of MI, and whether their destiny is already decided or can be modified. Do risk factors for MI coincide with those of atherosclerosis (ATS)? Is a positive family history of MI synonymous with genetic risk or do nongenetic familial factors also contribute to the overall familial risk? Can MI be considered a preventable event in subjects with a positive family history? Or, is the risk of the event already predetermined by the individual's genetic background, either as an additive effect of multiple low-dose contributors or as in monogenic diseases?

This article addresses the aforementioned questions regarding familiarity of MI, its risk factors, and genetics from a clinical perspective, to provide answers that can thus be applicable in the broader clinical context.

Funding sources: Dr Arbustini: National Ministry of Health "Ricerche Ricerche Correnti" 2005–2010 (IRCCS San Matteo, Pavia, Italy).
Conflict of Interest: Nil.
[a] Centre for Inherited Cardiovascular Diseases, Foundation IRCCS Policlinico San Matteo, P.le Golgi n. 19 27100 Pavia, Italy
[b] Institute of Cardiology, University of Bologna and S.Orsola-Malpighi Hospital, Via Massarenti 9, 40138 Bologna, Italy
[c] GVM Care and Research, presso Maria Cecilia Hospital, Via Corriera 1,48010 Cotignola, Italy
* Corresponding author. Centre for Heritable Cardiovascular Diseases, IRCCS Foundation Policlinico San Matteo, Piazzale Golgi 19, 27100 Pavia, Italy.
E-mail address: e.arbustini@smatteo.pv.it

Med Clin N Am 96 (2012) 67–86
doi:10.1016/j.mcna.2011.11.001
0025-7125/12/$ – see front matter © 2012 Elsevier Inc. All rights reserved.

---

**Key Points**

1. Although most risk factors for coronary atherosclerosis (ATS) (the rule) are also risk factors for myocardial infarction (MI) (the exception), MI-specific risk is likely additional to or independent from ATS risk. Recent genome-wide association studies have identified novel chromosomal loci with potential candidate genes that do not code for known risk factors, and thereby open new frontiers of research for MI-specific risk factors as well as novel biomarkers, unrelated with known risk factors. Endophenotypes, such as plasma levels or activity of gene products, could be more closely associated with genetic variations than is the eventual end phenotype (MI), which is a cumulative multifactorial event.

2. Because a positive family history for ATS risk factors does not fully coincide with a positive family history for MI, the risk stratification for MI should include family history data on number, age, and gender of affected family members, modifiable and nonmodifiable known risk factors, and unpredictable triggers.

3. Heritable factors playing a role in the coagulation, inflammatory, and adrenergic pathways, as well as associated epistatic and gene-environment interactions may be MI-specific contributors, but their individual role in MI cannot currently be translated, due to multilayered influences (by both genes and environment) on each factor.

4. Genetic counseling may contribute to implement family-tailored preventive strategies, taking into consideration the patient's clinical history, family history, and lifestyle. While waiting for genetic tests that add predictive contribution to the overall risk calculation, cardiologists can incorporate family history and clinical data to provide the best individualized monitoring and preventive programs. Although it cannot be ruled out that rare forms of monogenic MI exist, there is no evidence to date that MI is a monogenic disease.

5. Members from families with several affected relatives who have experienced MI should be reassured that their destiny is not predefined solely by the genetic ground, but that they simultaneously require family-specific protection.

---

## MI AND ATS RISK FACTORS PARTLY OVERLAP

Patients with different coronary ATS-related phenotypes are frequently grouped under the umbrella of coronary artery disease (CAD). However, in this setting MI is the exception[3] while its pathologic substrate ATS is the rule (**Fig. 1**).[4] Because the majority of MI occurs in individuals with coronary ATS, an obvious deduction is that risk factors are, at least partly, coincidental in ATS and MI. In daily practice, cardiologists cannot easily separate risk factors of MI from those of ATS, considering the contribution of: (1) non-modifiable factors, such as male gender, advanced age, exogenous acute triggers, and genetic make-up; (2) positive family history; and (3) known modifiable risk factors that include both those that are partly heritable and those that are exclusively exogenous (**Table 1**).[5–17]

Although it is now evident that genetic risk factors for MI do not fully coincide with those for ATS, large studies have reported that 9 known modifiable ATS risk factors account for greater than 90% of risk for an acute MI,[18] demonstrating that events and mortality can be prevented. Recent epidemiologic surveys reveal that control of risk factors in the United States over the last 4 decades have translated into lower incidence of coronary heart disease mortality, confirming that ongoing preventive strategies are effectively reaching the target, although hospitalization rates due to MI occurrence have stayed steady, owing to current diagnosis of MI making use of sensitive serum biomarkers.[19]

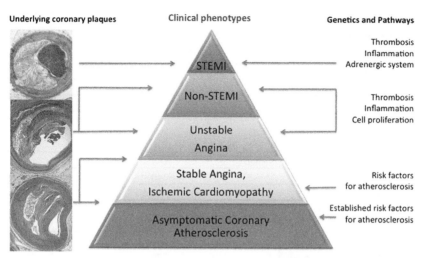

**Fig. 1.** Coronary artery disease is an umbrella term encompassing heterogeneous clinical phenotypes. Although the risk factors for myocardial infarction (MI) and atherosclerosis (ATS) partly overlap, MI is rare with respect to the more common coronary ATS. NSTEMI, non–ST-elevation MI; STEMI, ST-elevation MI.

## POSITIVE FAMILY HISTORY

Familial clustering of MI was well known before the development of molecular genetics.[20] A positive family history includes heritability and shared environmental risk factors. Specifically, heritability contributes to the multifactorial MI event, as it is the sum of several individual loci that, following the Mendelian rules of transmission, interact with the environment to predispose to or protect from the event.

Gender-related imprinting is a further contributor to familial risk of MI.[21] Although the more prevalent paternal family history of MI (81%), followed by maternal (32.4%) and biparental (13.4%) history,[22] may reflect the prevalence of MI in males, sex-specific interactions between proband and parents are present for family history of MI, with more stress required if maternal history of MI exists.[23] A gender-related parental effect has been also demonstrated for ATS risk factors including type 1 diabetes,[24] suggesting the involvement of imprinted genes on common metabolic risk factors.

The relative risk (RR) of MI is much higher in individuals with one or more affected first-degree relatives, with a higher RR when relatives are affected at earlier ages.[25] Specifically, in exploring positive fraternal history of MI, the relative hazard of coronary death was reported to be 13 times higher among monozygous male twins and 4 times higher among dizygous male twins, after one's twin died of premature CAD.[26] Although no more informative than sib pairs, dizygous twins have shared intrauterine life, and both ATS and related risk factors appear to originate during fetal life.[27] Twin studies thus provide substantial contributions to highlighting genetic factors, and can be beneficial in apportioning constituents of variance amongst genetic, and shared versus unique environmental, influences.[26,28] Nonetheless, family-related risk remains difficult to estimate in clinical practice because its contribution is subject to classification errors and bias, as well as descriptive ability and recall of participants; for example, daily clinical experience shows that the majority of sudden deaths (SD) that occur outside of the hospital setting are attributed by family members to MI, especially when autopsy is not performed, and therefore events such as pulmonary

**Table 1**
**Percentage of heritability of risk factors**

| Risk Factors | % Heritability | References |
|---|---|---|
| Nonmodifiable, Established | | |
| Male gender | — | — |
| Family history | 20–50 | 5 |
| Old age of affected family members carries lower risk for relatives and vice versa | — | 6 |
| Modifiable, Partly Heritable, Established | | |
| Diabetes mellitus, type 2 | 10 | 7 |
| Diabetes mellitus, type 2 | 40–80 | 6 |
| Diabetes mellitus, type 1 | 88 | 8 |
| Triglycerides | 40–80 | 6 |
| Increased LDL-cholesterol | 40–80 | 5 |
| LDL-cholesterol in young adult twins[a] | 79 | 9 |
| LDL-cholesterol in elderly twins | 18 | 10 |
| HDL | 45–75 | 6 |
| Total cholesterol | 40–60 | 6 |
| TC/HDL ratio | 49 | 11 |
| TG/HDL ratio | 39 | 11 |
| Hypertension | 50–70 | 5 |
| Obesity | 25–60 | 5 |
| Modifiable, Environmental, Established | | |
| Cigarette smoking | — | — |
| Lifestyle, sedentary | — | — |
| Stressful lifestyle | — | — |
| Behavioral and emotional individual make-up | — | — |
| Unpredictable, Exogenous, Nonmodifiable | | |
| Exogenous triggers | — | — |
| Heritable, Poorly Modifiable, Emerging | | |
| Lipoprotein(a) (90%) | 90 | 6 |
| Modifiable, Partly Heritable, Emerging | | |
| Small, dense LDL/atherogenic phenotype | 30–50 | 5 |
| Apolipoproteins A-I, C-II, C-III | 16–75 | 12 |
| Apolipoproteins A-II, B, E | 20–73 | 12 |
| Fibrinogen levels | 20–50 | 6 |
| Hyperhomocystinemia related to *MTHFR* | 45 | 6 |
| Plasma angiotensinogen (AGT) | 74[b] | 13 |
| C-reactive protein | 26–40 | 5 |
| Factors involved in metabolic syndrome | 16–40 | 5 |

(continued on next page)

| Table 1 (continued) | | |
|---|---|---|
| **Risk Factors** | **% Heritability** | **References** |
| Coronary artery calcifications | 40–50 | 5 |
| Partition of Heritability, Emerging | | |
| Plasminogen activator inhibitor-1 (PAI-1) | 42 | 14 |
| Cholesterol ester transfer protein (CETP) activity | Not available; modified by physical activity | 15 |
| Myeloperoxidase (MPO) | 23.8,[c] 25.1[d] | 16 |
| Cytokines: interleukins, IL-6 | 20.3,[c] 11.8[d] | 16 |
| Adiponectin | 39 | 17 |
| Leptin | 74 | 13 |

Most risk factors for ATS coincide with those recorded in patients with MI. Grouping heterotypes under the common umbrella of coronary artery disease associated with ATS has probably limited identification of MI-specific risk factors, or partitioning of the effects of risk factors shared by ATS and MI. The heritability values listed here have been retrieved from case examples in which the heritability of risk factors has been determined.

*Abbreviations:* ATS, atherosclerosis; HDL, high-density lipoprotein; LDL, low-density lipoprotein; MI, myocardial infarction; MTHFR, methylenetetrahydrofolate reductase; TC, total cholesterol; TG, triglycerides.

[a] Adjusted for body mass index.
[b] Depicts heritability of both male and female samples; plasma AGT heritability was different for male (89%) and female (53%) offspring samples.
[c] Age- and sex-adjusted.
[d] Multivariable-adjusted heritability, both with standard error of approximately 6%.

*Data from* Qasim A, Reilly MP. Genetic Determinants of Atherosclerotic Diseases. In Emery and Rimoin's Principles and Practice of Medical Genetics. 5th edition. Elsevier Health Sciences; 2006. p. 1334.

embolism, aortic dissection, and arrhythmogenic deaths are unlikely to be included in the differential. Further, no biomarker is currently measured for a highly relevant risk factor such as tobacco smoking (nicotinemia) or emotional triggers (catecholamine levels), eventually making it difficult to accurately partition the components of positive family history, family-related environment, and entirely exogenous factors.

## FAMILIAL ENVIRONMENTAL FACTORS

Family-related lifestyles and attitudes may contribute to familial risk factors. In broad terms the first quarter of an individual's life is spent within family, after which each individual may either conserve the familial lifestyle-associated "imprinting" or modify his or her habits.

### Diet

Well-balanced diets centered on plant foods improve health in comparison with meat-based diets, and have a favorable impact on CAD.[29] The intake of polyunsaturated fatty acids from fish is protective[30]; however, the estimated benefit may be confounded by association of methylmercury with MI.[31] Furthermore, salt consumption and hypertension, a strong risk factor for MI, are closely linked,[32] and individual taste, which is partially under genetic control,[33] may be influenced by the early use of salt. Dietary styles are therefore largely influenced by familial lifestyle-associated imprinting.

### Physical Activity

Regular, moderate to strenuous exercise is protective against acute MI,[18] and early childhood environmental factors importantly influence exercise levels throughout life. Monozygotic twin studies have documented long-term familial aggregation of adherence to exercise; a study of 117 adult monozygotic male twin pairs demonstrated considerable familial aggregation in exercise during adulthood, with 43% of total variation in exercise during adulthood constituted by familial aggregation.[34]

### Smoking and Education in the Family

Smoking constitutes a known risk factor for MI. Parental use of tobacco and reduced family cohesiveness are essential components of positive preteen attitudes toward smoking.[35] In a successfully followed cohort of more than 3000 children and parents, children having one parent who smokes raised their risk of becoming a daily smoker by 64% (odds ratio = 1.90, $P<.01$).[36]

### Familial Clustering of Infections

The association between MI and chronic infections caused by *Helicobacter pylori*, cytomegalovirus (CMV), *Chlamydia pneumoniae*, hepatitis viruses, or oral pathogens is still under investigation. These infections cluster in both families and institutions. The current hypothesis is that certain infections may play a role in vascular or systemic inflammation and therefore contribute to atherothrombosis.[37] Thus, the "infectious" familial risk of MI may contribute to a "positive" family history, or be an expression of genetic susceptibility to the infections.

## MI: LOW-DOSE INPUT OF MANY GENES

MI is one of the phenotypes associated with coronary ATS. The occurrence of MI in individuals without apparent risk factors highlights the existence of powerful yet still unknown risk factors that play their role independently of, or in addition to, the underlying coronary ATS.[38] However, most genetic research in the past has concentrated on CAD as a whole, often without distinction between different phenotypes; thus one frequently sees, gathered under the umbrella term CAD, series of patients with ST-elevation MI (STEMI) and non–ST-elevation MI (NSTEMI), as well as unstable or stable angina (see **Fig. 1**).

Novel studies are now beginning to distinguish MI and CAD as a whole; a recent genome-wide association study identified the novel 15q25.1 *ADAMTS7* locus in patients with angiographic CAD but no MI, and the 9q34.2 *ABO* locus in patients with both CAD and MI.[39] The contribution of genetics to CAD has been largely investigated, with replicated studies supporting the role of genes partaking in the coagulation or inflammatory pathways (discussed later), or of chromosomal loci in which unknown candidate genes map (reviewed in Ref.[40]), such as the 9p21.3 locus for CAD and MI identified via genome-wide association study, with over 30 independent study replicas (**Table 2**).[26,41–51]

## NOVEL CANDIDATE GENES, UNRELATED TO KNOWN RISK FACTORS, ADD TO CLASSIC RISK FACTORS

Most genes mapping in these new loci are widely distributed in the overall population, but they do not seem to be related to known risk factors, suggesting that novel pathogenetic pathways at still unexplored layers (including, eg, transcriptional factors) could contribute to the genetic risk of MI. Endophenotypes, such as plasma levels or activity of gene products, are likely more closely associated with genetic variations than are the genetic variations with the final phenotype, to which a given gene may be one of several contributors; thus, although the risk alleles are themselves not changed, targeting the gene products, for example, could modify their effects. This evidence constitutes the basis for emerging research on novel biomarkers (**Fig. 2**).

Excluding the role of potentially heritable known risk factors for ATS (see **Table 1**), heritable factors involved in coagulation, inflammatory and adrenergic pathways, and related epistatic and gene-environment interactions may be more specific players in the acute coronary event.

## The Coagulation Pathway

Several prothrombotic polymorphisms in genes encoding for factors involved in the coagulation cascade have been associated with MI predisposition (see, eg, Mendelian Inheritance in Man [MIM] +188039, Thrombomodulin; MIM *176929, Thrombin) or protection (MIM +134569, A subunit of factor XIII). In a recent meta-analysis on the factor V Leiden mutation (FVL), including 7790 MI cases and 19,276 controls, the presence of the FVL mutation was significantly greater in cases than in controls (6.791% vs 1.304%, respectively; odds ratio 1.608); the risk in individuals harboring FVL may have an effect on the genetic counseling of related family members for implementation of appropriate prophylactic measures.[52] However, most available data on other coagulation factors are still conflicting.

Many described variants map to different genes and loci, highlighting the low probability that a single individual carries all or several risky genetic variants. Prothrombotic variants of genes encoding coagulation factors are plausible candidates that may contribute to genetic risk of coronary thrombosis, although the recently documented contribution of hemorrhage to plaque core formation and complications[53] intriguingly suggests that the opposite hypothesis should also be considered.

## The Inflammatory Pathway

Due to the major role of inflammation in plaque destabilization and complication, genes encoding for inflammatory factors may contribute to MI-specific risk (MIM +153439, Lymphotoxin alpha; or MIM *603699, Arachidonate 5-lipoxygenase-activating protein). Furthermore, inflammatory and coagulation pathways are tightly linked and are subject to epistatic (gene-gene interactions, eg, allelic variants of thrombin-activated factor 2 receptor [F2R] that moderate interleukin [IL]-6 production[54]) and gene-environment interactions.

## The Adrenergic Pathway

The occurrence of MI in asymptomatic individuals subject to acute emotional or stressful triggers[2] raises the question as to whether the same individual would have developed MI in the absence of the acute trigger. The occurrence, albeit rare, of MI in patients with pheochromocytoma[55] strongly supports the role of catecholamines in MI. Polymorphisms of the human β1-adrenergic receptor genes (MIM +109689 -ADRB1, p.Arg389Gly [dbSNP:rs1801253]; MIM +10963 -ADRB2, p.Gln27Glu [dbSNP:rs1042714]) have also demonstrated an association with increased MI risk in some populations.

**Table 2**
Genome-wide association studies in CAD-MI identified novel disease loci and candidate genes; most of these latter do not code products related with classic risk factors

| Locus | SNP | No. of Cases | No. of Controls | Replicas | Gene and Function | Association | References |
|---|---|---|---|---|---|---|---|
| 1p13.1 | rs599839 linked to PSRC1 | 1231 MI | 560 | | Near SORT1 (Sortilin), a VPS10-containing receptor binding neuropeptides → Coreceptor of the p75-neurotrophin-receptor-mediated proapoptotic signal by pro-NGF | P-adjusted = .009 | 41 |
| | | 1926 CAD (WTCCC) | 2938 | German MI Family Study: 875 MI; 1644 controls | PSRC1 (Proline/Serine-Rich Coiled-Coil Protein 1) → Microtubule-interacting and -bundling protein with prosurvival function | $P = 4.05 \times 10^{-9a}$ | 42 |
| | | 11,550 CAD; 59% MI | 11,205 | | | $P = 1.44 \times 10^{-7}$ for CAD | 43,b |
| | rs646776 linked to CELSR2 | 2967 early-onset MI | 3075 | Independent sample = 19,492 | CELSR2 (Cadherin EGF LAG seven-pass G-type receptor 2) → Participate in cell adhesion and receptor-ligand interactions | $P = .04$ | 44 |
| 1p32 | rs11206510 Not located in known genes | | | | Near PCSK9 (Proprotein Convertase, Subtilisin/Kexin-Type, 9) → Decreases hepatic and extrahepatic LDL receptor levels, increases plasma LDL-cholesterol levels | $P = .02$ | 44 |
| 1q41 | rs17465637 linked to MIA3 | 1926 CAD (WTCCC) | 2938 | German MI Family Study: 875 MI; 1644 controls | Near MIA3 (Melanoma Inhibitory Activity Protein 3 → Necessary for loading bulky trimeric collagen VII molecules into transport vesicles for secretion. Also referred to as TANGO1 | $P = 1.27 \times 10^{-6a}$ | 42 |
| | rs3008621 | 11,550 CAD; 59% MI | 11,205 | | | $P = 1.02 \times 10^{-3}$ for CAD | 43 |
| | rs17465637 | 1231 MI | 560 | | | P-adjusted = 0.0034 | 41 |
| | rs17465637 | 2967 early-onset MI | 3075 | Independent sample = 19,492 | | $P = 1.5 \times 10^{-4}$ | 44 |

| Locus | SNP | Sample 1 | Sample 2 | Study | Gene/Function | P value | Ref |
|---|---|---|---|---|---|---|---|
| 2q36.3 | rs2943634 Not located in known genes | 1926 CAD (WTCCC) | 2938 | German MI Family Study: 875 MI; 1644 controls | Intergenic | $P = 1.19 \times 10^{-5}$ | 42 |
| | | 11,550 CAD; 59% MI | 11,205 | | | $P = 3.22 \times 10^{-2}$ for CAD[c] | 43,b |
| 2q33 | rs6725887 linked to WDR12 | 2967 | 3075 | Independent sample = 19,492 | WDR12 (WD-repeat-containing protein 12 (WD = Trp-Asp) → Involved in cell cycle progression, signal transduction, apoptosis, (ribosome biogenesis protein) | $P = 8.6 \times 10^{-5}$ | 44 |
| 3q22.3 | rs9818870 linked to MRAS | 1222 German MI | 1298 | 3 genome-wide CAD datasets and replication in ~25,000 subjects | MRAS (Muscle RAS Oncogene Homolog) → Membrane-anchored guanosine-5'-triphosphate–binding protein → intracellular signal transducers | $P = 2.38 \times 10^{-5}$ | 45 |
| 6p24 | rs12526453 linked to PHACTR1 | 2967 | 3075 | Independent sample = 19,492 | PHACTR1 (Phosphatase and Actin Regulator 1) → Protein phosphatase inhibitor, binds actin | $P = 4.6 \times 10^{-4}$ | 44 |
| 6q26-27 | rs2048327, linked to SLC22A3 rs3127599 linked to LPAL2 rs7767084 and rs10755578 linked to LPA | 1926 CAD (WTCCC) | 2938 | 8999 cases and 10,263 controls, including WTCCC study. Strong global haplotypic association adjusted for study ($P = 1.34 \times 10^{-21}$) | SLC22A3 → Important participant in elimination of endogenous small organic cations, drugs, and environmental toxins LPAL2 → C-terminally truncated compared with apolipoprotein(a) LPA (apolipoprotein(a)) | $P = 4.34 \times 10^{-8}$ for haplotype association | 46 |
| | rs10455872 and rs3798220 linked to LPA | 3145 | 3352 | 4846 CAD and 4594 controls (from PROCARDIS trios, ISIS study, SHEEP, SCARF) | LPA (apolipoprotein(a)) | Association with rs10455872: $P = 3.4 \times 10^{-15}$ | 47 |

(continued on next page)

**Table 2**
**(continued)**

| Locus | SNP | No. of Cases | No. of Controls | Replicas | Gene and Function | Association | References |
|---|---|---|---|---|---|---|---|
| 6q25.1 | rs6922269 linked to MTHFD1L | 1926 CAD (WTCCC) | 2938 | German MI Family Study: 875 MI; 1644 controls | MTHFD1L Methylenetetrahydrofolate dehydrogenase (NADP+-dependent) 1-like protein → Participates in tetrahydrofolate synthesis in mitochondria | $P = 6.33 \times 10^{-6}$ | 42 |
| | | 11,550 CAD; 59% MI | 11,205 | | | $P = 1.96 \times 10^{-2}$ for CAD[c] | 43 |
| 9p21.3 | rs2383207 (correlated with rs10116277 and rs1333040) Not located in known genes | 1607 Icelandic MI | 6728 | 665 Icelandic MI 3533 controls + 3 case-control sample sets of European descent | Near CDKN2A and CDKN2B CDKN2A. Tumor suppressor locus → somatic mutation, deletion, or silencing in pancreatic cancer, glioma, and melanoma | $P = 1.4 \times 10^{-6}$ | 48 |
| | rs10757274 rs2383206 | 322 CHD | 312 | 311 cases and 326 controls (OHS-2), 1347 cases and 9054 controls (ARIC).[d] | CDKN2B. Encodes a cyclin-dependent kinase inhibitor → regulates G1 progression in cell cycle | For rs10757274: $P = 3.7 \times 10^{-6}$ For rs2383206: $P = 6.7 \times 10^{-6}$. | 49 |
| | rs1333049 | 1926 CAD (WTCCC) | 2938 | German MI Family Study: 875 MI; 1644 controls | | $P = 1.80 \times 10^{-14}$ | 42 |
| | | 11,550 CAD; 59% MI | 11,205 | | | $P = 2.89 \times 10^{-21}$ for CAD | 43,b |
| | rs4977574 | 2967 | 3075 | Independent sample = 19,492 | | $P = 6.7 \times 10^{-9}$ | 44 |
| 9q34.2 | ABO | 5783 CAD with MI | 3644 CAD but no MI | | ABO: Glycosyltransferase catalyzes carbohydrate transfer onto the H antigen of red blood cells to form the A or B antigens | $P = 7.62 \times 10^{-9}$ | 26 |

| 10q11.21 | rs501120 Not located in known gene | 1926 CAD (WTCCC) | 2938 | German MI Family Study: 875 MI; 1644 controls | Near CXCL12 (Chemokine, CXC Motif, Ligand 12) → Stromal cell-derived alpha chemokine → activates lymphocytes and is involved in metastasis of certain cancers, including breast | $P = 9.46 \times 10^{-8a}$ | 42 |
|---|---|---|---|---|---|---|---|
| | | 11,550 CAD; 59% MI | 11,205 | | " | $P = 4.34 \times 10^{-4}$ for CAD. In women: $P = 1.86 \times 10^{-5}$ | 43,b |
| 10q11 | rs1746048 Not located in known gene | 2967 | 3075 | Independent sample = 19,492 | Near CXCL12 (Chemokine, CXC Motif, Ligand 12) | $P = 1.6 \times 10^{-4}$ | 44 |
| 12q24.31 | rs2259816 linked to HNF1A | 1222 German | 1298 | 3 genome-wide CAD datasets and replication in ~25,000 subjects | Near -HNF1A (Hepatocyte Nuclear Factor 1 alpha) → Transcriptional factor that regulates expression and function of a variety of hepatocyte-specific genes. -C12orf43 (Chromosome 12 open reading frame 43) → Uncharacterized | $P = 2 \times 10^{-4}$ | 45 |
| 12q24 | rs3184504 linked to SH2B3 | 2625 Icelandic discovery | 33,625 | 4025 cases, 6996 controls: combined replication in 6 datasets of European descent | SH2B3 (SH2B adaptor protein 3) → Mediates the interaction between extracellular receptors and intracellular signaling pathways, important role in hematopoiesis | $P = .0012$ | 50 |
| 15q24.2 | ADAMTS7 | 12,393 CAD without MI | 7383 no CAD | | ADAMTS7 (A Disintegrin And Metalloproteinase with Thrombospondin Motifs 7) | $P = 4.98 \times 10^{-13}$ | 26 |

(continued on next page)

**Table 2**
*(continued)*

| Locus | SNP | No. of Cases | No. of Controls | Replicas | Gene and Function | Association | References |
|---|---|---|---|---|---|---|---|
| 15q22.33 | rs17228212 linked to *SMAD3* | 1926 CAD (WTCCC) | 2938 | German MI Family Study: 875 MI; 1644 controls | *SMAD3* → Signal transducer and transcriptional modulator, involved in carcinogenesis regulation | $P = 1.98 \times 10^{-7a}$ | [42] |
| | rs17228212 | 11,550 CAD; 59% MI | 11,205 | Locus did not replicate | | $P = .893$ for CAD | [43] |
| 19p13 | rs1122608 linked to *SMARCA4* | 2967 | 3075 | Independent sample = 19,492 | Near *LDLR* → low-density lipoprotein receptor | $P = 1.7 \times 10^{-4}$ | [44] |
| 21q22 | rs9982601 Not located in known gene | 2967 | 3075 | Independent sample = 19,492 | Near -*MRPS6* (Mitochondrial Ribosomal Protein S6) → -28S subunit protein of the ribosomal protein S6P family. -*SLC5A3* (Solute Carrier Family 5 Inositol Transporter Member 3 → Involved in *myo*-inositol transport. -*KCNE2* (Potassium channel, Voltage-gated; ISK-related Subfamily member 2) → -*LQT6* gene | $P = 7.8 \times 10^{-4}$ | [44] |
| 22q12.1 | rs2301523 Not located in known gene | 188 Japanese MI patients | 752 Japanese | 3464 MI patients, 3819 controls: general population | *MIAT* (myocardial infarction associated transcript) → 4 MIAT variants may function as RNAs; in vitro translation → no protein products | $P = .0006$ | [51] |

*Abbreviation:* WTCCC, Wellcome Trust Case Control Consortium.
[a] Combined analysis of WTCCC and German MI Family Study.
[b] Samani, et al. report that these loci acted independently and cumulatively increased CAD risk by 15% (12%–18%), per additional risk allele.
[c] Not statistically significant after correction for multiple testing.
[d] Validation in 2326 cases and 10,427 controls (Copenhagen City Heart Study, Dallas Heart Study, Ottawa Heart Study–3).

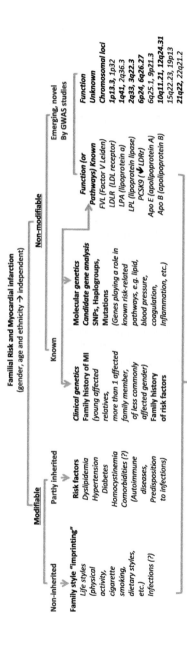

**Fig. 2.** Familial risk and myocardial infarction. A schematic of modifiable and nonmodifiable factors contributing to the acute event. SNP, single-nucleotide polymorphism.

### Gene-Environment Interactions

Individuals who are genetically predisposed to MI (positive family history) but not exposed to acute or chronic environmental risk factors may not develop MI, and vice versa. Genetic predictors of minor risk in the overall population may predict a high risk in specific subsets of individuals as a result of the interaction between the gene and environmental factor (including cigarette smoking, infections, meals, and drugs) or gender (see **Fig. 2**).[6]

## MONOGENIC FACTORS

Autosomal dominant MI has been associated with mutations in the Myocyte-specific Enhancer Factor-2 (*MEF2A)* gene (*ADCAD1*, MIM #608319).[56] The MIM symbol # indicates that the associated phenotype is described and the molecular bases are known, as in monogenic disorders. Assuming a monogenic inheritance, a positive linkage (log odds ratio = 4.19) was found to map to a single locus (*adCAD1*) on chromosome 15q26, and a 21-bp coding sequence deletion in an evolutionarily conserved region of *MEF2A* (MIM *600659), cosegregated with the phenotype in affected relatives.[56] Shortly afterward, however, the deletion was not confirmed as being associated with CAD/MI.[57] Although the association remains under debate and the presence of other rare Mendelian forms of CAD cannot be ruled out, the *MEF2A* gene example underscores the possibility that emerging risk factors may not have known measurable intermediate biochemical or clinical traits.

## NEXT-GENERATION SEQUENCING

Next-generation sequencing (NGS) tools are progressive, lowering of the costs for whole genome scans, and will soon generate challenge strategies of risk stratification based on individual-specific genome-wide analysis. While at present querying Online MIM for genetic susceptibility of MI reveals 182 entries, sequencing the entire genome will provide identification of numerous single-nucleotide polymorphisms (SNPs) and copy number variations per individual of known, uncertain, and unknown function and relevance.

A recent report on a single 40-year-old man underwent genome-wide sequencing that identified genetic variants associated with increased risk of MI as well as other monogenic and multifactorial diseases, including sudden cardiac death, type 2 diabetes, and some cancers.[58] The evolution of whole-genome individual sequencing will require novel strategies of data analysis and interpretation, as it will reveal multilayered levels of risk for numerous monogenic and multifactorial diseases. Because whole-genome sequencing is still restricted to a few and selected applications because of the high costs, exome sequencing, which analyzes the protein-coding portion of the genome, is closer to clinical translation and places many advantages of the emerging technologies into researchers' hands.[59] Indeed, a recent "targeted evidence-based review based on published Evaluation of Genomic Applications in Practice and Prevention methodologies" showed that even if novel genomic markers are independent of traditional risk factors, cardiovascular disease risk reclassification would be small.[60]

## KNOWN RISKY ALLELES AND PERSONAL RISK STRATIFICATION IN CURRENT CLINICAL PRACTICE

The potential predictive value of MI-specific risky alleles should be considered either independently of family history or in the context of a positive family history, especially when risky alleles segregate with the phenotype in the family. Within families, risky alleles could indicate a higher genetic risk than in the general population of unrelated individuals. Given the high number of risky alleles and their high frequency in the general population, and considering that each SNP is associated with a small positive effect, the majority of the carrier population is expected to be exposed to an increased genetic risk. Accordingly, even a small genetic contribution may increase the overall prevalence of MI. However, until protective alleles are also fully elucidated, the calculation of the genetic risk based on genetic testing will show only one side of the coin.

An open question is whether risk alleles exert synergistic effects, and this question is unlikely to be clarified before elucidation of MI-related effects of risky alleles or identification of novel biomarkers that measure intermediate products or endophenotypes related to the function of novel candidate genes or loci. When asked about novel genetic tests for predicting MI, cardiologists should let patients know about the recent progression of research and that SNP-based predicting assays do exist, but are far from being scientifically proven as additional to, or more contributory than, an informative positive family history.

## ROLE OF GENETIC COUNSELING

An important goal of genetic counseling with family pedigree construction is the establishment of tailored preventive strategies based on the patient's clinical history, family history, lifestyle, and attitudes. The scenarios vary in different families, as shown in **Fig. 3**, and the compilation of information from family screening, including cardiologic and biochemical assessment of risk factors, will be beneficial. Distinguishing positive family history for risk factors from positive family history for MI is essential to dissect the percentage of known modifiable risk factors from nonmodifiable factors. When counseling a family member whose parent(s) or sibling(s) have experienced MI, the individual's likelihood to develop MI should be calculated considering the additive effects of:

- Nonmodifiable risk factors, such as gender, age, and family history of MI, as well as acute emotional triggers, chronic stress, or multiple adverse life events
- All-inclusive positive family history of MI, including both heritable and shared environmental factors
- Age and gender of affected relatives versus age of unaffected family members exposed to the risk; the risk in relatives of patients with premature MI is higher because genetic influences decline in the elderly who carry the cumulative impact of environmental factors
- The positive family history for risk factors and pattern of inheritance of risk factors, such as diabetes and hypercholesterolemia, among others, in the family, and the RR of each risk factor on MI
- The interaction of genetic and environmental factors (and the worsening effects of external factors in the case of genetic predisposition).

Although the impact of unpredictable risk cannot be measured, familial risk can be graded as high or low by integrating simple and low-cost data. Accordingly, an individual can be predicted to be at highest risk based on family history, if more than one relative is affected and if the affected relative is closely related, has experienced premature MI, or is of the less commonly affected gender (see **Fig. 3**). Thus, an absolute risk score cannot be generated, but risk can be estimated to be low, medium, or high using these key criteria, keeping in mind that high individual variability exists. Clinical family screening in premature MI with more than one affected family member

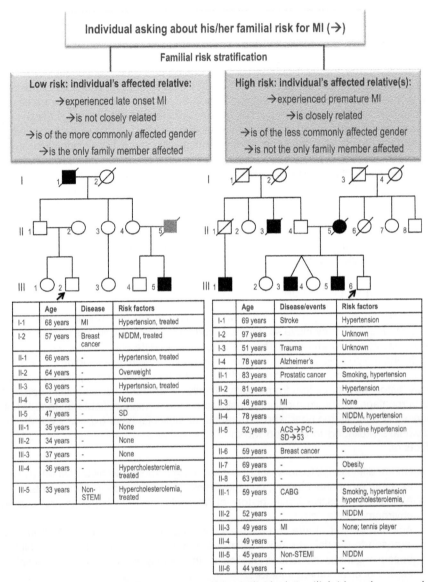

**Fig. 3.** Assessing familial risk for MI in an inquiring individual. Familial risk can be assessed as high or low using the criteria elucidated in the figure, keeping in mind that there exists considerable variability between the two. Family member III-2 of the low-risk pedigree asked for counseling after the acute event in his cousin (III-5). However, the closest affected relative in his family is his paternal grandfather, who developed MI at the age of 68 years. It is very possible that the acute event in III-5 could have been influenced by his paternal (II-5) rather than maternal lineage. Family member III-6 of the high-risk pedigree asked for genetic counseling after the acute event of his younger brother (III-3). His mother suffered acute coronary syndrome 1 year before sudden death, and 2 of his brothers experienced acute ischemic events. The highest risk can be estimated for the female twin and the male brother who are clinically healthy. The 3 healthy siblings should undergo regular clinical monitoring and receive education and guidance regarding healthy lifestyles. ACS, acute coronary syndrome; CABG, coronary artery bypass graft; MI, myocardial infarction; NIDDM, non–insulin-dependent diabetes mellitus; PCI, percutaneous coronary intervention; SD, sudden death; STEMI, ST-elevation myocardial infarction.

could thus be the first step in family-tailored preventive strategies to be implemented in clinical practice.

## SUMMARY

Although a positive family history does constitute a significant risk factor for MI, MI occurrence depends on the multifaceted interplay between genetic and environmental factors. Thus, familial clustering of MI should not merely be considered a synonym of heritability, but rather a combination of inherited and environmental factors (some of which are shared by family members), keeping in mind that lifestyle is a highly subjective matter and that control of known risk factors lowers the risk.

While waiting clinical translation of genetic testing in risk stratification, relatives alerted by an MI in a family member should receive tailored stratification of familial risk, and be reassured that offspring of parents experiencing premature MI do not necessarily have a 50% risk of developing MI as adults because MI, with few and still debated exceptions, remains a multifactorial disease.

## REFERENCES

1. Finn AV, Nakano M, Narula J, et al. Concept of vulnerable/unstable plaque. Arterioscler Thromb Vasc Biol 2010;30:1282–92.
2. Bhattacharyya MR, Steptoe A. Emotional triggers of acute coronary syndromes: strength of evidence, biological processes, and clinical implications. Prog Cardiovasc Dis 2007;49:353–65.
3. Bertomeu A, García-Vidal O, Farré X, et al. Preclinical coronary atherosclerosis in a population with low incidence of myocardial infarction: cross sectional autopsy study. Br Med J 2003;327:591–2.
4. Arbustini E, Grasso M, Diegoli M, et al. Coronary thrombosis in noncardiac death. Coron Artery Dis 1993;4:751–9.
5. Qasim A, Reilly MP. Genetic Determinants of Atherosclerotic Diseases. In Emery and Rimoin's Principles and Practice of Medical Genetics. 5th edition. Elsevier Health Sciences; 2006. p. 1334. Accessed September 10, 2011.
6. Lusis AJ, Mar R, Pajukanta P. Genetics of atherosclerosis. Annu Rev Genomics Hum Genet 2004;5:189–218.
7. Billings LK, Florez JC. The genetics of type 2 diabetes: what have we learned from GWAS? Ann N Y Acad Sci 2010;1212:59–77.
8. Hyttinen V, Kaprio J, Kinnunen L, et al. Genetic liability of type 1 diabetes and the onset age among 22,650 young Finnish twin pairs: a nationwide follow-up study. Diabetes 2003;52:1052–5.
9. Pietiläinen KH, Söderlund S, Rissanen A, et al. HDL subspecies in young adult twins: heritability and impact of overweight. Obesity (Silver Spring) 2009;17:1208–14.
10. Rahman I, Bennet AM, Pedersen NL, et al. Genetic dominance influences blood biomarker levels in a sample of 12,000 Swedish elderly twins. Twin Res Hum Genet 2009;12:286–94.
11. Isaacs A, Sayed-Tabatabaei FA, Aulchenko YS, et al. Heritabilities, apolipoprotein E, and effects of inbreeding on plasma lipids in a genetically isolated population: the Erasmus Rucphen Family Study. Eur J Epidemiol 2007;22:99–105.
12. Cai YP, Hayakawa K, Nishihara R, et al. Heritability of serum apolipoprotein concentrations in middle-aged Japanese twins. J Epidemiol 2009;19:260–5.

13. Watkins WS, Rohrwasser A, Peiffer A, et al. AGT genetic variation, plasma AGT, and blood pressure: an analysis of the Utah Genetic Reference Project pedigrees. Am J Hypertens 2010;23:917–23.
14. Hong Y, Pedersen NL, Egberg N, et al. Moderate genetic influences on plasma levels of plasminogen activator inhibitor-1 and evidence of genetic and environmental influences shared by plasminogen activator inhibitor-1, triglycerides, and body mass index. Arterioscler Thromb Vasc Biol 1997;17: 2776–82.
15. Ahmad T, Chasman DI, Buring JE, et al. Physical activity modifies the effect of LPL, LIPC, and CETP polymorphisms on HDL-C levels and the risk of myocardial infarction in women of European ancestry. Circ Cardiovasc Genet 2011;4: 74–80.
16. Schnabel RB, Lunetta KL, Larson MG, et al. The relation of genetic and environmental factors to systemic inflammatory biomarker concentrations. Circ Cardiovasc Genet 2009;2:229–37.
17. Liu PH, Jiang YD, Chen WJ, et al. Genetic and environmental influences on adiponectin, leptin, and BMI among adolescents in Taiwan: a multivariate twin/sibling analysis. Twin Res Hum Genet 2008;11:495–504.
18. Yusuf S, Hawken S, Ounpuu S, et al. Effect of potentially modifiable risk factors associated with myocardial infarction in 52 countries (the INTERHEART study): case-control study. Lancet 2004;364:937–52.
19. Parikh NI, Gona P, Larson MG, et al. Long-term trends in myocardial infarction incidence and case fatality in the National Heart, Lung, and Blood Institute's Framingham Heart study. Circulation 2009;119:1203–10.
20. Rose G. Familial patterns in ischaemic heart disease. Br J Prev Soc Med 1964;18: 75–80.
21. Sesso HD, Lee IM, Gaziano JM, et al. Maternal and paternal history of myocardial infarction and risk of cardiovascular disease in men and women. Circulation 2001;104:393–8.
22. Greenlund KJ, Valdez R, Bao W, et al. Verification of parental history of coronary artery disease and associations with adult offspring risk factors in a community sample: the Bogalusa Heart Study. Am J Med Sci 1997;313:220–7.
23. Banerjee A, Silver LE, Heneghan C, et al. Sex-specific familial clustering of myocardial infarction in patients with acute coronary syndromes. Circ Cardiovasc Genet 2009;2:98–105.
24. McCann JA, Xu YQ, Frechette R, et al. The insulin-like growth factor-II receptor gene is associated with type 1 diabetes: evidence of a maternal effect. J Clin Endocrinol Metab 2004;89:5700–6.
25. Roncaglioni MC, Santoro L, D'Avanzo B, et al. Role of family history in patients with myocardial infarction. An Italian case-control study. GISSI-EFRIM Investigators. Circulation 1992;85:2065–72.
26. Marenberg ME, Risch N, Berkman LF, et al. Genetic susceptibility to death from coronary heart disease in a study of twins. N Engl J Med 1994;330:1041–6.
27. Palinski W, Napoli C. The fetal origins of atherosclerosis: maternal hypercholesterolemia, and cholesterol-lowering or antioxidant treatment during pregnancy influence in utero programming and postnatal susceptibility to atherogenesis. FASEB J 2002;16:1348–60.
28. Hunter DJ. Gene-environment interactions in human diseases. Nat Rev Genet 2005;6:287–98.
29. Sabaté J. The contribution of vegetarian diets to health and disease: a paradigm shift? Am J Clin Nutr 2003;78:502S–7S.

30. Mozaffarian D, Ascherio A, Hu FB, et al. Interplay between different polyunsaturated fatty acids and risk of coronary heart disease in men. Circulation 2005;11: 157–64.

31. Stern AH. A review of the studies of the cardiovascular health effects of methylmercury with consideration of their suitability for risk assessment. Environ Res 2005;98:133–42.

32. Lev-Ran A, Porta M. Salt and hypertension: a phylogenetic perspective. Diabetes Metab Res Rev 2005;21:118–31.

33. Garcia-Bailo B, Toguri C, Eny KM, et al. Genetic variation in taste and its influence on food selection. OMICS 2009;13:69–80.

34. Simonen RL, Videman T, Kaprio J, et al. Factors associated with exercise lifestyle—a study of monozygotic twins. Int J Sports Med 2003;24:499–505.

35. Bush T, Curry SJ, Hollis J, et al. Preteen attitudes about smoking and parental factors associated with favorable attitudes. Am J Health Promot 2005;19: 410–7.

36. Peterson AV Jr, Leroux BG, Bricker J, et al. Nine-year prediction of adolescent smoking by number of smoking parents. Addict Behav 2006;31:788–801.

37. Anderson JL, Muhlestein JB. The role of infection. In: Theroux P, editor. Acute coronary syndromes: a companion to Braunwald's heart disease. Philadelphia: Saunders; 2003. p. 88–107.

38. Zimmerman FH, Cameron A, Fisher LD, et al. Myocardial infarction in young patients: Angiographic characterization, risk factors and prognosis (Coronary Artery Surgery Registry). J Am Coll Cardiol 1995;26:654–61.

39. Reilly MP, Li M, He J, et al. Identification of ADAMTS7 as a novel locus for coronary atherosclerosis and association of ABO with myocardial infarction in the presence of coronary atherosclerosis: two genome-wide association studies. Lancet 2011;377:383–92.

40. Musunuru K, Kathiresan S. Genetics of coronary artery disease. Annu Rev Genomics Hum Genet 2010;11:91–108.

41. Wang AZ, Li L, Zhang B, et al. Association of SNP rs17465637 on chromosome 1q41 and rs599839 on 1p13.3 with myocardial infarction in an American Caucasian population. Ann Hum Genet 2011;75:475–82.

42. Samani NJ, Erdmann J, Hall AS, et al. Genome-wide association analysis of coronary artery disease. N Engl J Med 2007;357:443–53.

43. Samani NJ, Deloukas P, Erdmann J, et al. Large scale association analysis of novel genetic loci for coronary artery disease. Arterioscler Thromb Vasc Biol 2009;29:774–80.

44. Kathiresan S, Voight BF, Purcell S, et al. Genome-wide association of early-onset myocardial infarction with single nucleotide polymorphisms and copy number variants. Nat Genet 2009;41:334–41.

45. Erdmann J, Grosshennig A, Braund PS, et al. New susceptibility locus for coronary artery disease on chromosome 3q22.3. Nat Genet 2009;41:280–2.

46. Trégouët DA, König IR, Erdmann J, et al. Genome-wide haplotype association study identifies the SLC22A3-LPAL2-LPA gene cluster as a risk locus for coronary artery disease. Nat Genet 2009;41:283–5.

47. Clarke R, Peden JF, Hopewell JC, et al. Genetic variants associated with Lp(a) lipoprotein level and coronary disease. N Engl J Med 2009;361:2518–28.

48. Helgadottir A, Thorleifsson G, Manolescu A, et al. A common variant on chromosome 9p21 affects the risk of myocardial infarction. Science 2007;316:1491–3.

49. McPherson R, Pertsemlidis A, Kavaslar N, et al. A common allele on chromosome 9 associated with coronary heart disease. Science 2007;316:1488–91.

50. Gudbjartsson DF, Bjornsdottir US, Halapi E, et al. Sequence variants affecting eosinophil numbers associate with asthma and myocardial infarction. Nat Genet 2009;41:342–7.
51. Ishii N, Ozaki K, Sato H, et al. Identification of a novel non-coding RNA, MIAT, that confers risk of myocardial infarction. J Hum Genet 2006;51:1087–99.
52. Dowaidar M, Settin A. Risk of myocardial infarction related to factor V Leiden mutation: a meta-analysis. Genet Test Mol Biomarkers 2010;14:493–8.
53. Michel JB, Virmani R, Arbustini E, et al. Intraplaque haemorrhages as the trigger of plaque vulnerability. Eur Heart J 2011;32:1977–85.
54. Gigante B, Vikström M, Meuzelaar LS, et al. Variants in the coagulation factor 2 receptor (F2R) gene influence the risk of myocardial infarction in men through an interaction with interleukin 6 serum levels. Thromb Haemost 2009;101:943–53.
55. Garg A, Banitt PF. Pheochromocytoma and myocardial infarction. South Med J 2004;97:981–4.
56. Wang L, Fan C, Topol SE, et al. Mutation of MEF2A in an inherited disorder with features of coronary artery disease. Science 2003;302:1578–81.
57. Weng L, Kavaslar N, Ustaszewska A, et al. Lack of MEF2A mutations in coronary artery disease. J Clin Invest 2005;115:1016–20.
58. Ashley EA, Butte AJ, Wheeler MT, et al. Clinical assessment incorporating a personal genome. Lancet 2010;375:1525–35.
59. Majewski J, Schwartzentruber J, Lalonde E, et al. What can exome sequencing do for you? J Med Genet 2011;48:580–9.
60. Palomaki GE, Melillo S, Neveux L, et al. Use of genomic profiling to assess risk for cardiovascular disease and identify individualized prevention strategies—a targeted evidence-based review. Genet Med 2010;12:772–84.

# Age As a Risk Factor

Ravi Dhingra, MD, MPH[a], Ramachandran S. Vasan, MD, DM[b,c,*]

KEYWORDS

• Age • Cardiovascular disease • Risk

*It is not by the gray of the hair that one knows the age of the heart.*
—*Edward Bulwer-Lytton*

According to the most recent estimates from the United States, cardiovascular disease (CVD) death rates have declined but the disease burden remains substantially high.[1] The risk of developing CVD is largely (75–90%) explained by the presence or absence of traditional CVD risk factors.[2] Age is a well-known traditional risk factor, which is generally considered nonmodifiable for obvious reasons. This review discusses the common use of an individual's age in prediction of CVD incidence using different risk scores, examines whether or not age as a risk factor can be modified, discusses the methods used to evaluate long-term and short-term CVD risk, addresses appropriate communication of an individual's risk based on age group and CVD risk, and concludes by discussing the influence of age on cardiac and vascular risk factors.

## ASSESSMENT OF CVD RISK USING AGE AS PART OF RISK SCORES

With aging, there is an incremental acquisition of several CVD risk factors in an individual's lifespan. When these risk factors are incorporated in a multivariable regression model, age remains an independent risk factor. There are several risk prediction scores currently available to assess an individual's risk of CVD, and all of them include age as a predictor. Older age, as assessed by these risk scores, is associated with greater risk of CVD.

Disclosures: none.

This work was supported by contract NO1 25195 from the National Institutes of Health.

[a] Section of Cardiology, Dartmouth Medical School, Heart and Vascular Center, Dartmouth-Hitchcock Medical Center, One Medical Center Drive, Lebanon, NH 03756, USA

[b] Section of Preventive Medicine and Epidemiology, Department of Medicine, Boston University School of Medicine, Boston, MA, USA

[c] The Framingham Heart Study, 73 Mount Wayte Avenue, Suite 2, Framingham, MA 01702-5803, USA

* Corresponding author. The Framingham Heart Study, 73 Mount Wayte Avenue, Suite 2, Framingham, MA 01702-5803.

*E-mail address:* vasan@bu.edu

Although there are several risk scores available, the Framingham risk score (FRS)[3] is one of the most widely adopted screening tools in United States and is recommended by National Heart, Lung, and Blood Institute to assess an individual's CVD risk.[4,5] Other risk scores, which are tested in Britain,[6] Scotland,[7] New Zealand,[8] or China,[9] have not been formally tested in the United States. In addition to the traditional risk factors (age, gender, smoking, total cholesterol, high-density lipoprotein [HDL] cholesterol, and systolic blood pressure, which are part of the FRS), risk scores developed in Britain and Scotland incorporate family history and social deprivation as risk factors, and these additional variables marginally improve prediction of CVD risk over the FRS when applied to the British and the Scottish populations, respectively. The Reynolds risk score also includes age as a component and is constructed using a database of middle-aged American women and requires the additional measurements of C-reactive protein and hemoglobin $A_{1c}$ (in diabetics).[10] Lastly, the risk prediction score reported in prior European studies[11] and currently adopted by the joint European societies[12] is based on models that predict CVD death and, therefore, underestimates the burden of CVD by not including the nonfatal events. Although CVD death rates have declined in some developed European countries (similar to the trend in the United States), the overall CVD burden remains high.

## AGE IS AN INDEPENDENT RISK FACTOR FOR CARDIOVASCULAR DISEASE

As discussed previously, even after adjusting for traditional risk factors in a multivariable CVD prediction model, age remains a fundamental predictor of CVD risk. When age and other risk factors are used jointly to examine an individual's future risk of CVD, however, it has been postulated that the contribution of age in the multivariable models may be a reflection of the intensity and the duration of exposure to other traditional CVD risk factors.[13] If this observation were true, avoidance of these other risk factors should result in a reduction of CVD risk associated with age per se. To examine this hypothesis, prior studies from Framingham Heart Study have shown that the absence of each of these traditional risk factors is associated with a reduction in the risk of CVD even at an older age.[14] When the absence of multiple risk factors is factored into an individual's CVD risk assessment, the reduction in CVD risk is further augmented. Similarly, using the Framingham cohort, investigators have observed that lower midlife blood pressure and total cholesterol levels, absence of glucose intolerance, smoking abstinence, higher education, and female gender all predicted increased survival up to 85 years of age.[15] Additionally, at an older age, the contribution of age to CVD risk prediction declines, in part because there is less time left for individuals to acquire other modifiable CVD risk factors. Therefore, age at any given point influences the assessment of both short-term and long-term CVD risks of individuals. The absence of these CVD risk factors not only prevents the development of CVD but also decreases the risk of age-associated comorbidities and mortality.[15] In another prior study, after excluding individuals with cancer, CVD, or diabetes before 50 years of age, investigators followed the Framingham cohort to evaluate who was likely to reach 75 years of age. They concluded that smoking fewer cigarettes per day, lower systolic blood pressure, and higher forced vital capacity were associated with longevity in both genders.[16] Moreover, these observations relating to presence and absence of traditional risk factors have also been confirmed in a population-based study in the Japanese cohort from the Honolulu Heart Program,[17] and the large-scale, multiethnic, and international INTERHEART Study.[18] The INTERHEART Study investigators also tested this hypothesis in a case-control fashion among all age groups and observed similar results for prevention of myocardial infarction.[18] Therefore, it is well established that life expectancy of individuals is dependent on modification of traditional risk factors, and age-associated risk of CVD can be minimized by correcting or avoidance of these risk factors. Risk factor modification, however, is equally important for both young and older individuals and decreases their subsequent risk of CVD.

## RELATIVE RISK VERSUS ABSOLUTE RISK ASSESSMENT

Current CVD risk assessment using the FRS comprises the traditional risk factors (ie, cholesterol [total and HDL], blood pressure, history of smoking, and age).[3,5] When assessing risk of CVD, both short-term (10-year CVD risk) and long-term (>10 year) risks for CVD should be evaluated and communicated appropriately to individuals.[19] At a younger age, individuals with several CVD risk factors (ie, smoking, increased cholesterol, and high blood pressure) have a lower absolute short-term risk (compared with older individuals with similar CVD risk factors), and the absolute risk increases as the person gets older. The relative risk, however, remains relatively invariant throughout a person's lifespan provided other risk factors (except age) do not change, and it may decrease over time. Similarly, older individuals with several risk factors have a higher short-term absolute risk (compared with younger individuals with a similar risk factor profile) even though the relative risk may remain constant through the lifespan, provided there is no change in risk factors.

## COMMUNICATING CVD RISK TO YOUNG AND OLD

Communicating short-term or long-term CVD risks to patients can be challenging and might overestimate or underestimate the importance of risk factor reduction and, therefore, have an impact on how a person reacts by changing lifestyle for future risk reduction. For example, communicating an overestimated relative risk to young individuals might result in emotional or financial stress (may require them to take medications) whereas communicating an underestimated absolute risk may result in a lower level of motivation on the part of individuals to work toward changing their lifestyle to reduce CVD risk.[20]

Current guidelines from the Adult Treatment Panel III for treatment of high blood cholesterol appropriately incorporates both relative risk and absolute risk assessment aspects (discussed previously) for individuals and provides flexibility for discussion by a treating physician in primary prevention settings.[4,5] Prior investigators have cautioned treating physicians to distance themselves from communicating the magnified relative risk of individuals (compared with lower absolute risk) to achieve professionally desirable goals.[20]

## INFLUENCE OF AGE ON OTHER INDIVIDUAL RISK FACTORS

It is intuitive that if age is an independent risk factor for developing CVD, the lifetime risk of CVD for individuals would continue to increase with age. The lifetime risk for CVD, however, is lower at age 70 than at age 50 years for individuals whose lifestyle risk factors remain unchanged.[14] Similarly, lifetime risk of coronary artery disease,[21] stroke,[22] hypertension,[23] and heart failure[24] does not continue to increase with age. One explanation for this observation is that there is a shorter time period left for older individuals to develop the disease and a greater hazard of death due to competing causes. Other reasons are that those who live longer have inherent bias of lower burden of cardiovascular risk factors, which lowers their risk of developing an event, or a genetic makeup with resistance to developing CVD. The Framingham cohort enrolled individuals at their midlife (30–62 y) primarily but the INTERHEART study included some young participants (<40 y) and both showed similar results that reduction or absence of risk factors is additive and improves mortality. Consequently, screening for risk factors and advice about modifications of risk factors should start at an early age.

## INFLUENCE OF INDIVIDUAL RISK FACTORS ON AGE-ASSOCIATED CVD RISK

A gender-specific analysis from the Framingham cohort suggests that approximately 11.9% (men) to 40.3% (women) of age-associated CVD risk may be attributable to the concomitant burden of other CVD risk factors.[25] These estimates are based on comparing unadjusted regression coefficients for age with those obtained after adjusting for other CVD risk factors in multivariable models (systolic blood pressure, diabetes, total cholesterol to HDL cholesterol ratio, history of smoking, and body mass index).

## SUMMARY

The risk of developing CVD is generally dependent on the presence or absence of traditional risk factors. Increasing age is an independent risk factor for CVD, however. The burden of CVD risk associated with rising age can be reduced partly by the modification of traditional coexisting CVD risk factors. When communicating an individual's CVD risk regardless of age, short-term (10-year) and long-term (>10 years) risks (both absolute and relative risks) should be discussed and the subsequent management of CVD risk factors individualized.

## REFERENCES

1. Roger VL, Go AS, Lloyd-Jones DM, et al. Heart disease and stroke statistics—2011 update: a report from the American Heart Association. Circulation 2011; 123:e18–209.
2. Vasan RS, Sullivan LM, Wilson PW, et al. Relative importance of borderline and elevated levels of coronary heart disease risk factors. Ann Intern Med 2005; 142:393–402.
3. D'Agostino RB, Vasan RS, Pencina MJ, et al. General cardiovascular risk profile for use in primary care. Circulation 2008;117:743–53.
4. Expert Panel on Detection, Evaluation, and Treatment of High Blood Cholesterol in Adults. Executive Summary of the Third Report of the National Cholesterol Education Program (NCEP) Expert Panel on Detection, Evaluation, and Treatment of High Blood Cholesterol in Adults (Adult Treatment Panel III). JAMA 2001;285: 2486–97.
5. Grundy SM, Cleeman JI, Merz CN, et al. Implications of Recent Clinical Trials for the National Cholesterol Education Program Adult Treatment Panel III Guidelines. Circulation 2004;110:227–39.
6. Hippisley-Cox J, Coupland C, Vinogradova Y, et al. Derivation and validation of QRISK, a new cardiovascular disease risk score for the United Kingdom: prospective open cohort study. BMJ 2007;335:136.
7. Woodward M, Brindle P, Tunstall-Pedoe H. Adding social deprivation and family history to cardiovascular risk assessment: the ASSIGN score from the Scottish Heart Health Extended Cohort (SHHEC). Heart 2007;93:172–6.
8. Jackson R. Updated New Zealand cardiovascular disease risk-benefit prediction guide. BMJ 2000;320:709–10.

9. Zhang XF, Attia J, D'Este C, et al. A risk score predicted coronary heart disease and stroke in a Chinese cohort. J Clin Epidemiol 2005;58:951–8.

10. Ridker PM, Buring JE, Rifai N, et al. Development and validation of improved algorithms for the assessment of global cardiovascular risk in women. JAMA 2007;297:611–9.

11. Conroy RM, Pyörälä K, Fitzgerald AP, et al. Estimation of ten-year risk of fatal cardiovascular disease in Europe: the SCORE project. Eur Heart J 2003;24: 987–1003.

12. Graham I, Atar D, Borch-Johnsen K, et al. European guidelines on cardiovascular disease prevention in clinical practice: executive summary. Eur Heart J 2007;28: 2375–414.

13. Sniderman AD, Furberg CD. Age as a modifiable risk factor for cardiovascular disease. Lancet 2008;371:1547–9.

14. Lloyd-Jones DM, Leip EP, Larson MG, et al. Prediction of lifetime risk for cardio-vascular disease by risk factor burden at 50 years of age. Circulation 2006;113: 791–8.

15. Terry DF, Pencina MJ, Vasan RS, et al. Cardiovascular risk factors predictive for survival and morbidity-free survival in the oldest-old framingham heart study participants. J Am Geriatr Soc 2005;53:1944–50.

16. Goldberg RJ, Larson M, Levy D. Factors associated with survival to 75 years of age in middle-aged men and women: the Framingham study. Arch Intern Med 1996;156:505–9.

17. Willcox BJ, He Q, Chen R, et al. Midlife risk factors and healthy survival in men. JAMA 2006;296:2343–50.

18. Yusuf S, Hawken S, Ôunpuu S, et al. Effect of potentially modifiable risk factors associated with myocardial infarction in 52 countries (the INTERHEART study): case-control study. Lancet 2004;364:937–52.

19. Vasan RS, D'Agostino RB. Age and time need not and should not be eliminated from the coronary risk prediction models. Circulation 2005;111:542–5.

20. Epstein RM, Alper BS, Quill TE. Communicating evidence for participatory deci-sion making. JAMA 2004;291:2359–66.

21. Lloyd-Jones DM, Larson MG, Beiser A, et al. Lifetime risk of developing coronary heart disease. Lancet 1999;353:89–92.

22. Seshadri S, Beiser A, Kelly-Hayes M, et al. The lifetime risk of stroke. Stroke 2006; 37:345–50.

23. Vasan RS, Beiser A, Seshadri S, et al. Residual lifetime risk for developing hyper-tension in middle-aged women and men. JAMA 2002;287:1003–10.

24. Lloyd-Jones DM, Larson MG, Leip EP, et al. Lifetime risk for developing conges-tive heart failure. Circulation 2002;106:3068–72.

25. Kannel WB, Vasan RS. Is age really a non-modifiable cardiovascular risk factor? Am J Cardiol 2009;104:1307–10.

# Coronary Artery Disease in Aging Women: A Menopause of Endothelial Progenitor Cells?

Randolph Hutter, MD[a],*, Juan Jose Badimon, PhD[a],
Valentin Fuster, MD, PhD[a,b], Jagat Narula, MD, PhD[a]

---

**KEYWORDS**

- Coronary artery disease • Women • Atherogenesis
- Endothelium

---

## THE EMERGING ROLE OF ENDOTHELIAL PROGENITOR CELLS IN ATHEROGENESIS

The health of the vasculature is critically dependent on the integrity and appropriate functional activity of the luminal endothelium. A cascade of pathophysiologic events all originating at the endothelium as the interface between blood and vascular wall is involved in the process of atherogenesis and ultimately results in the development and progression of atherosclerotic lesions.[1–3] This process is well delineated for clinical vascular disease in humans and in multiple experimental animal models. A variety of different cardiovascular risk factors all exert their damaging effect on the arterial wall initially by the induction of endothelial injury. The ensuing endothelial expression of adhesion molecules leads to inflammatory events, with monocytes infiltrating the arterial wall and triggering smooth muscle cell proliferation resulting in the formation of atherosclerotic lesions.[3] Also during later and more advanced stages of atherosclerosis, luminal endothelial integrity is an important defense mechanism to prevent disease progression via atherosclerotic plaque erosion and rupture causing myocardial infarction and sudden cardiovascular death.[1,4] For all these reasons, the ability to maintain endothelial integrity despite an adverse risk factor profile is of crucial importance.

Traditionally, the repair of the luminal endothelium has been thought to originate from proliferation and migration of local resident and fully differentiated endothelial cells in analogy to the process of neovascularization (**Fig. 1**). Multiple studies have identified a population of presumably bone marrow–derived cells, labeled circulating

---

[a] Mount Sinai School of Medicine, 1 Gustave L. Levy Place, Box 1030, New York, NY 10029-6574, USA
[b] Fundación Centro Nacional de Investigaciones Cardiovasculares Carlos III, Melchor Fernández Almagro, 3, E-28029 Madrid, Spain
* Corresponding author.
*E-mail address:* Randolph.Hutter@mssm.edu

Med Clin N Am 96 (2012) 93–102
doi:10.1016/j.mcna.2012.01.008
0025-7125/12/$ – see front matter © 2012 Elsevier Inc. All rights reserved.

medical.theclinics.com

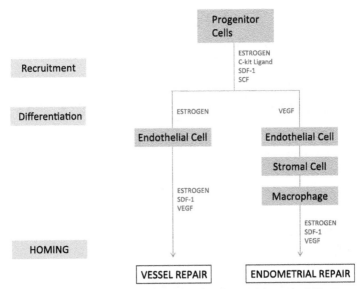

**Fig. 1.** Process from progenitor cells to vessel and endometrial repair. SCF, stem cell factor; SDF-1, stromal cell-derived factor-1; VEGF, vascular endothelial growth factor. (*Data from* Sata M. Role of circulating vascular progenitor cells in angiogenesis, vascular healing, and pulmonary hypertension: lessons from animal models. Arterioscler Thromb Vasc Biol 2006;26:1008–14.)

endothelial progenitor cells (EPCs), which can be isolated from bone marrow or circulating peripheral blood-derived, mononuclear cells.[5,6] These cells express multiple different surface markers attributed to endothelial cells, they incorporate into sites of neovascularization, and adhere to damaged luminal endothelial surfaces, thereby selectively homing to sites of vascular injury.[7–11]

Several clinical studies showed that the numbers of circulating EPCs are modulated by the presence of cardiovascular risk factors and that the functional state of the endothelium correlates with the functional state of EPCs.[12,13] The peripheral blood EPCs act as a circulating pool of cells capable of maintaining the critical homeostasis of the luminal endothelial vascular surface. In addition, EPCs are mobilized from bone marrow to peripheral blood by ischemic events, home to the ischemic tissues, and stimulate local angiogenesis. Reduced levels of circulating EPCs have been shown with increased classic risk factors for cardiovascular disease; however, more importantly, a scarcity of EPC has been shown to predict future adverse cardiovascular events. Therefore, EPCs may be considered to be a key cardiovascular defense mechanism as well as a potential novel biomarker that indicates cardiovascular health.[12–17]

## UNIQUE FEMALE CARDIOVASCULAR PROTECTION DURING THE REPRODUCTIVE AGE

Cardiovascular disease ranks as a leading cause of morbidity and mortality of women in the Western world, and the incidence of coronary events in women is still increasing, with most occurring after the onset of menopause.[18] It is thought that declining levels of endogenous estrogen in conjunction with age and the higher prevalence of obesity and altered body fat distribution result in a proatherogenic metabolic environment and the development of significant vascular endothelial dysfunction.[19–21]

Despite the significant increase in cardiovascular morbidity and mortality in post-menopausal women, the direct causal relationship between a lack of estrogen after menopause and the increased cardiovascular risk is still debated. The higher prevalence of traditional cardiovascular risk factors such as hypertension, hyperglycemia, and the presence of endothelial dysfunction among postmenopausal women might be related to the increased cardiovascular risk rather than a direct effect of estrogen deficiency.[19–21]

Premature menopause of natural and surgical cause has been linked to an increased cardiovascular risk compared with a timely menopause pointing to a cumulative protective effect of estrogen over the lifetime in women.[22,23] Several effects of estrogen could be relevant to the observed cardiovascular protection over the lifetime. These effects include estrogen actions on ventricular contractile function, coronary calcification processes, effects on endothelial calcium metabolism, on decreased insulin resistance, oxidative alterations of lipids, and changes in overall lipid profile.[24–27]

Two estrogen receptor isoforms are known, ER-$\alpha$ and ER-$\beta$, with both being expressed in cardiovascular cells and tissues.[28] Estrogen receptors belong to a class of receptors with ligand-induced activation of transcription factors and subsequent changes in gene expression. This receptor behavior is categorized as genomic and is responsible for most of the long-term effects of estrogens. In addition, nongenomic mechanisms exist and do not depend on changes in gene expression. One important example of this mode of estrogen action is the activation of endothelial nitric oxide synthase leading to arterial vasodilation after administration of estrogens.[28]

Despite all this evidence and the results of observational studies suggesting that postmenopausal hormone replacement therapy could lower cardiovascular risk,[29] randomized placebo-controlled trials have shown no benefit for postmenopausal estrogen replacement therapy, but instead show adverse effects on cardiac and thromboembolic events.[30]

Some investigators point out that the time window between onset of menopause and the start of hormone replacement therapy might be at the core of these discrepant findings suggesting that the longer an estrogen deficient state lasted, the greater the lack of benefit, or even the incidence of detrimental effects with hormone replacement therapy.[31]

Contrary to the conceptual contradictions surrounding postmenopausal hormone replacement therapy, the important finding remains that women at the reproductive age exhibit a significantly lower cardiovascular risk than age-matched men.[32] This is generally attributed to the differences in sex hormones and, specifically, to the protective properties of female estrogens for the cardiovascular system described earlier.[28,33] Available data suggest that the protective cardiovascular properties of the female hormonal status might be achieved by modulating EPC function.[34,35]

## EXAMINING THE OBVIOUS: WHAT IS UNIQUE ABOUT THE FEMALE ENDOTHELIAL PROGENITOR CELL BIOLOGY DURING THE REPRODUCTIVE AGE?

To address the question about what features are unique in the EPC biology of women of reproductive age, the question of what is unique about the female reproductive system in general must be addressed.

In the female reproductive system, angiogenic events are a key component and recurrent feature in the setting of cyclical buildup and repair of endometrial tissue.[36] The interplay between systemic ovarian sex steroid hormones and the local endometrial response determines the profound changes in tissue composition and remodeling during the menstrual cycle. Estrogen and progesterone coordinate alternating uterine cell proliferation with enhanced neovascularization and subsequent tissue regression/destruction. Several studies suggest that this synchronized angiogenic process in the endometrium is mediated by direct hormonal regulation of the local expression of angiogenic growth factors.[37–40]

Traditionally, this angiogenic activity in the uterus was thought to be accomplished by the proliferation and migration of fully differentiated endothelial cells via sprouting from parent vessels, consistent with the concept of classic angiogenesis.[41] More recently, increasing evidence suggests vasculogenesis rather than angiogenesis to occur in reproductive organs. Vasculogenesis is defined as the incorporation of circulating EPCs derived from the bone marrow into neovascularization foci and has been described in adult species in multiple settings.[5,7]

The circulating EPCs are clearly linked to endometrial vascular turnover,[42] and the systemic pretreatment with estrogen in several experimental models enhances EPC mobilization as measured by a culture assay; it may also augment neovascularization in mouse cornea. Moreover, using bone marrow transplant experiments with transfer of bone marrow from tie-2 GFP–expressing mice into wild-type mice, the authors showed the incorporation of tie-2 GFP–expressing EPC into estrogen-stimulated endometrium in conjunction with increased local vascular endothelial growth factor (VEGF) expression. This finding adds an important aspect to the incorporation of other blood-borne cells such as macrophages into the endometrial stroma as shown by earlier reports. In posthuman HLA/sex-mismatched bone marrow transplantation, 14% of endometrial endothelial cells and 50% of stromal cells were derived from the newly transplanted bone marrow and not from the recipient's parenchymal cells, strongly suggesting that endometrial vasculogenesis also occurs in humans.[42–44]

There is also evidence of estrogen regulating bioactivity of EPC showing increase in steady-state EPC after hysterectomy in rats, as measured by sca-1+ and CD31+ cells.[42] A similar direct effect of the ovarian hormonal regulation over the process of vasculogenesis in the adult has been shown in the setting of luminal endothelial repair when EPCs incorporate into the endothelial lining during reendothelialization after arterial injury. In this setting, estrogen significantly enhanced the incorporation of EPC and accelerated luminal endothelial repair in a fashion comparable with VEGF therapy.[45,46]

However, the definition of truly angiogenic circulating EPC remains controversial. Several publications suggest that CD34+/KDR+ EPC best correlates with cardiovascular risk and subclinical atherosclerosis. Several other marker combinations have been used to identify and quantify EPCs, as well as the approach of detecting colony-forming units of EPC from peripheral blood mononuclear cells instead of fluorescent cell sorting analysis. This lack of standardization has resulted in difficulty comparing results from one EPC study with another.[47–49]

These methodological issues might also contribute to the discussion surrounding conflicting data generated by a recent small study showing an increase in circulating EPCs in postmenopausal women, again illustrating methodological challenges in determining identity, number, and function of EPCs. This study stands in contrast with studies equating differential gender risk for cardiovascular disease after menopause with decreased EPC numbers and function in women after menopause.[34]

Therefore, some investigators challenge the approach of measuring colony formation of EPCs as an inferior method compared with fluorescence activated cell sorting analysis, which again reflects the overlap and difficult distinction between circulating EPCs and monocyte/macrophage-derived cells.[35,50] Significant menstrual modulation has not been observed with all different types of EPC and this suggests selective properties of certain EPC populations in their involvement in endometrial turnover and their responsiveness to female sex hormones such as estrogen.[51,52]

Another approach to solving the dilemma of choosing the best EPC detection method is to put the emphasis on angiogenic and functional characteristics of EPCs in vitro and in in vivo models rather than mere expression of endothelial cell–like markers using mainly the expression of e-NOS to differentiate between true late EPCs and monocytic EPCs, and then to test the cells for their angiogenic potential.[53,54]

What remains undisputable is that, in the blood of women during active reproductive cycling, a higher number of endothelial colonies can be found and that there is increased adherence of female EPC to damaged endothelium and increased angiogenesis in rat ischemic muscle in vivo.[55–58]

Equally evident is that mobilization of EPCs occurs during hormonal cycles and that certain EPC are clearly influenced by female sex hormones. In animals with estrogen deficiency after ovariectomy, a reduction in the number of circulating EPCs was observed, resulting in impaired reendothelialization after carotid injury that was reversible with exogenous estrogen replacement.[46,58]

The physiologic control of EPCs by estrogens occurs at multiple levels such as EPC differentiation, proliferation, migration, apoptosis, as well as incorporation and mobilization.[42] There occurs a significant variation in the numbers and the morphology of EPCs during the menstrual cycle of healthy female volunteers, and an enhanced differentiation potential of circulating EPCs after peak estrogen levels during the menstrual cycle.[42] With peak estrogen levels, an increased expression of vascular endothelial cadherin and KDR/flk-VEGF receptor was seen on EPC, consistent with an essential function of these molecules described during embryonic vasculogenesis.[59–62]

The range of effects of 17-β estradiol extended from a suppression of neointima formation to a modulation of the telomerase activity of EPCs, thereby enhancing their repair potential.[58,63,64] As shown by several groups, functional estrogen receptors are key in regulating EPC bioactivity. This finding has been studied on the mRNA and protein expression level, using specific receptor-blockade, ER-α, and ER-β knockout mice. It seems that the ER-α isoform is more relevant for vasculogenesis occurring under pathologic conditions and that the ER-β isoform of the receptor is more relevant for physiologic vasculogenesis.[42,55] Moreover, male EPCs seem more responsive to the mitogenic effects of estrogen than female EPCs, which possess a higher level of stimulation already at baseline, consistent with a constitutive activation of estrogen receptor signaling in female EPC. Nonselective and α-selective inhibition of estrogen receptor function result in reduced EPC generation and decreased adhesion of these cells. Conversely, when comparing male versus female EPCs derived from cord blood, ER-β activity prevailed in male EPCs compared with female, with the 2 isoforms acting antagonistically regarding their biologic effects in EPC.[65]

Several groups have not found a clear cyclic pattern of VEGF levels or a coordinated change in the expression of VEGF receptors on EPCs or in the endometrium during the menstrual cycle,[66–68] which leads to the question of whether other key regulatory molecules of the angiogenic process are altered during different phases of the menstrual cycle, or whether the observed differences in EPC biology are solely mediated by estrogen. Therefore, it is of great interest that, in ovulatory women, EPC number and soluble c-kit ligand levels vary in a coordinated fashion during the menstrual cycle. C-kit ligand is cleaved by MMP-9 activity in the bone marrow induced by stromal cell–derived factor-1 (SDF-1)–and linked to the mobilization of cells from the bone marrow, which in turn have been shown to integrate into the endometrial lining in humans.[69–71] Another important regulator of EPC biology is SDF-1, which facilitates mobilization and extravasation of EPCs through changes in their integrin expression. In addition, SDF-1 has been shown to enhance stem cell homing and to induce differentiation of EPCs.[72–75]

Several groups report a significant increase in systemic levels of SDF-1 during the proliferative phase of the menstrual cycle as opposed to increased local expression of SDF in the endometrium during the secretory phase. Consistent with these data, an inverse relationship between colony formation of EPC and systemic SDF levels was reported, pointing to SDF-1 as an extravasation signal that depletes the number of circulating EPC. During the secretory phase, SDF-1 levels were lower and EPC numbers were significantly higher.[76,77] Other myeloid mobilizing molecules such as colony-stimulating factor (CSF) and granulocyte-macrophage CSF that have been shown to mobilize EPC could not be detected in healthy female volunteers with active reproductive cycles during the menstrual cycle.[76]

## LESSONS TO BE LEARNED

The cardiovascular protection provided to women during the reproductive age and the unique angiogenic properties of the female reproductive system provide insights into how angiogenesis, EPC biology, and atherogenesis are intertwined in a complex regulatory network of female sex hormones, angiogenic growth factors, and stem cell regulatory molecules. Hormone replacement therapy after menopause,[31] attempts at proangiogenic therapies during myocardial and vascular injury,[78,79] as well as more recent attempts at bone marrow stem cell/EPC therapy,[80–81] show that the sole modulation of a single component does not yield clinical success or sufficient impact on the underlying biology. The intricate and interwoven endometrial physiology of the female menstrual cycle linking systemic factors (hormones, angiogenic growth factors, stem cell regulatory molecules), bone marrow and circulating bone marrow–derived cells, and local endometrial growth factor expression/cell homing makes it clear that, to harness the physiologic cardioprotection provided by nature to women of reproductive age for better cardiovascular therapies in postmenopausal women and the population in general, a more coherent and systematic approach is needed than has previously been used.

Plaque erosion is thought to be the basis of acute coronary syndromes in premenstrual women with smoking usually as the only coronary risk factor.[82] It seems that the protective effect of EPC seeding may be nullified by smoking. Inconclusive trends of increased late stent thrombosis after drug-eluting stent placement in smokers may also allude to long-term impairment of endothelial healing.

## REFERENCES

1. Badimon JJ, Zaman A, Helft G, et al. Acute coronary syndromes: pathophysiology and preventive priorities. Thromb Haemost 1999;82:997–1004.
2. Fuster V, Fayad ZA, Badimon JJ. Acute coronary syndromes: biology. Lancet 1999;353(Suppl 2):SII5–9.
3. Libby P, Ridker PM, Maseri A. Inflammation and atherosclerosis. Circulation 2002; 105:1135–43.
4. Burke AP, Farb A, Malcom GT, et al. Coronary risk factors and plaque morphology in men with coronary disease who died suddenly. N Engl J Med 1997;336:1276–82.
5. Asahara T, Murohara T, Sullivan A, et al. Isolation of putative progenitor endothelial cells for angiogenesis. Science 1997;275:964–7.
6. Rafii S, Meeus S, Dias S, et al. Contribution of marrow-derived progenitors to vascular and cardiac regeneration. Semin Cell Dev Biol 2002;13:61–7.

7. Asahara T, Masuda H, Takahashi T, et al. Bone marrow origin of endothelial progenitor cells responsible for postnatal vasculogenesis in physiological and pathological neovascularization. Circ Res 1999;85:221–8.
8. Fujiyama S, Amano K, Uehira K, et al. Bone marrow monocyte lineage cells adhere on injured endothelium in a monocyte chemoattractant protein-1-dependent manner and accelerate reendothelialization as endothelial progenitor cells. Circ Res 2003; 93:980–9.
9. Griese DP, Ehsan A, Melo LG, et al. Isolation and transplantation of autologous circulating endothelial cells into denuded vessels and prosthetic grafts: Implications for cell-based vascular therapy. Circulation 2003;108:2710–5.
10. Takahashi T, Kalka C, Masuda H, et al. Ischemia- and cytokine-induced mobilization of bone marrow-derived endothelial progenitor cells for neovascularization. Nat Med 1999;5:434–8.
11. Walter DH, Rittig K, Bahlmann FH, et al. Statin therapy accelerates reendothelialization: a novel effect involving mobilization and incorporation of bone marrow-derived endothelial progenitor cells. Circulation 2002;105:3017–24.
12. Rosenzweig A. Circulating endothelial progenitors–cells as biomarkers. N Engl J Med 2005;353:1055–7.
13. Werner N, Nickenig G. Influence of cardiovascular risk factors on endothelial progenitor cells: limitations for therapy? Arterioscler Thromb Vasc Biol 2006;26:257–66.
14. Hristov M, Erl W, Weber PC. Endothelial progenitor cells: mobilization, differentiation, and homing. Arterioscler Thromb Vasc Biol 2003;23:1185–9.
15. Schmidt-Lucke C, Rossig L, Fichtlscherer S, et al. Reduced number of circulating endothelial progenitor cells predicts future cardiovascular events: proof of concept for the clinical importance of endogenous vascular repair. Circulation 2005;111:2981–7.
16. Urbich C, Dimmeler S. Endothelial progenitor cells: characterization and role in vascular biology. Circ Res 2004;95:343–53.
17. Werner N, Kosiol S, Schiegl T, et al. Circulating endothelial progenitor cells and cardiovascular outcomes. N Engl J Med 2005;353:999–1007.
18. Ouyang P, Michos ED, Karas RH. Hormone replacement therapy and the cardiovascular system lessons learned and unanswered questions. J Am Coll Cardiol 2006;47:1741–53.
19. Berg G, Mesch V, Boero L, et al. Lipid and lipoprotein profile in menopausal transition. Effects of hormones, age and fat distribution. Horm Metab Res 2004;36:215–20.
20. Matthan NR, Jalbert SM, Lamon-Fava S, et al. TRL, IDL, and LDL apolipoprotein B-100 and HDL apolipoprotein A-I kinetics as a function of age and menopausal status. Arterioscler Thromb Vasc Biol 2005;25:1691–6.
21. Shimabukuro M, Higa N, Asahi T, et al. Fluvastatin improves endothelial dysfunction in overweight postmenopausal women through small dense low-density lipoprotein reduction. Metabolism 2004;53:733–9.
22. Hu FB, Grodstein F, Hennekens CH, et al. Age at natural menopause and risk of cardiovascular disease. Arch Intern Med 1999;159:1061–6.
23. Mondul AM, Rodriguez C, Jacobs EJ, et al. Age at natural menopause and cause-specific mortality. Am J Epidemiol 2005;162:1089–97.
24. Ayres S, Abplanalp W, Liu JH, et al. Mechanisms involved in the protective effect of estradiol-17beta on lipid peroxidation and DNA damage. Am J Physiol 1998; 274:E1002–8.
25. Ren J, Hintz KK, Roughead ZK, et al. Impact of estrogen replacement on ventricular myocyte contractile function and protein kinase B/Akt activation. Am J Physiol Heart Circ Physiol 2003;284:H1800–7.

26. Strehlow K, Rotter S, Wassmann S, et al. Modulation of antioxidant enzyme expression and function by estrogen. Circ Res 2003;93:170–7.
27. Sumino H, Ichikawa S, Itoh H, et al. Hormone replacement therapy decreases insulin resistance and lipid metabolism in Japanese postmenopausal women with impaired and normal glucose tolerance. Horm Res 2003;60:134–42.
28. Mendelsohn ME, Karas RH. The protective effects of estrogen on the cardiovascular system. N Engl J Med 1999;340:1801–11.
29. Davidson MH, Testolin LM, Maki KC, et al. A comparison of estrogen replacement, pravastatin, and combined treatment for the management of hypercholesterolemia in postmenopausal women. Arch Intern Med 1997;157:1186–92.
30. Rossouw JE, Anderson GL, Prentice RL, et al. Risks and benefits of estrogen plus progestin in healthy postmenopausal women: principal results from the women's health initiative randomized controlled trial. JAMA 2002;288:321–33.
31. Rossouw JE, Prentice RL, Manson JE, et al. Postmenopausal hormone therapy and risk of cardiovascular disease by age and years since menopause. JAMA 2007;297:1465–77.
32. Wenger NK. Coronary heart disease: an older woman's major health risk. BMJ 1997;315:1085–90.
33. Cignarella A, Paoletti R, Puglisi L. Direct effects of estrogen on the vessel wall. Med Res Rev 2001;21:171–84.
34. Bulut D, Albrecht N, Imohl M, et al. Hormonal status modulates circulating endothelial progenitor cells. Clin Res Cardiol 2007;96:258–63.
35. Hoetzer GL, MacEneaney OJ, Irmiger HM, et al. Gender differences in circulating endothelial progenitor cell colony-forming capacity and migratory activity in middle-aged adults. Am J Cardiol 2007;99:46–8.
36. Reynolds LP, Killilea SD, Redmer DA. Angiogenesis in the female reproductive system. FASEB J 1992;6:886–92.
37. Ferrara N, Chen H, Davis-Smyth T, et al. Vascular endothelial growth factor is essential for corpus luteum angiogenesis. Nat Med 1998;4:336–40.
38. Goede V, Schmidt T, Kimmina S, et al. Analysis of blood vessel maturation processes during cyclic ovarian angiogenesis. Lab Invest 1998;78:1385–94.
39. Losordo DW, Isner JM. Estrogen and angiogenesis: a review. Arterioscler Thromb Vasc Biol 2001;21:6–12.
40. Shweiki D, Itin A, Neufeld G, et al. Patterns of expression of vascular endothelial growth factor (VEGF) and VEGF receptors in mice suggest a role in hormonally regulated angiogenesis. J Clin Invest 1993;91:2235–43.
41. Folkman J, Klagsbrun M. Angiogenic factors. Science 1987;235:442–7.
42. Masuda H, Kalka C, Takahashi T, et al. Estrogen-mediated endothelial progenitor cell biology and kinetics for physiological postnatal vasculogenesis. Circ Res 2007;101:598–606.
43. Bonatz G, Hansmann ML, Buchholz F, et al. Macrophage- and lymphocyte-subtypes in the endometrium during different phases of the ovarian cycle. Int J Gynaecol Obstet 1992;37:29–36.
44. Fernandez-Shaw S, Clarke MT, Hicks B, et al. Bone marrow-derived cell populations in uterine and ectopic endometrium. Hum Reprod 1995;10:2285–9.
45. Hutter R, Carrick FE, Valdiviezo C, et al. Vascular endothelial growth factor regulates reendothelialization and neointima formation in a mouse model of arterial injury. Circulation 2004;110:2430–5.
46. Iwakura A, Luedemann C, Shastry S, et al. Estrogen-mediated, endothelial nitric oxide synthase-dependent mobilization of bone marrow-derived endothelial progenitor cells contributes to reendothelialization after arterial injury. Circulation 2003;108:3115–21.

47. Fadini GP, Avogaro A, Agostini C. Critical assessment of putative endothelial progenitor phenotypes. Exp Hematol 2007;35:1479–80 [author reply: 1481–2].
48. Fadini GP, Coracina A, Baesso I, et al. Peripheral blood CD34+KDR+ endothelial progenitor cells are determinants of subclinical atherosclerosis in a middle-aged general population. Stroke 2006;37:2277–82.
49. Fadini GP, de Kreutzenberg SV, Coracina A, et al. Circulating CD34+ cells, metabolic syndrome, and cardiovascular risk. Eur Heart J 2006;27:2247–55.
50. Prater DN, Case J, Ingram DA, et al. Working hypothesis to redefine endothelial progenitor cells. Leukemia 2007;21:1141–9.
51. Madeddu P, Emanueli C, Pelosi E, et al. Transplantation of low dose CD34+KDR+ cells promotes vascular and muscular regeneration in ischemic limbs. FASEB J 2004;18:1737–9.
52. Pelosi E, Valtieri M, Coppola S, et al. Identification of the hemangioblast in postnatal life. Blood 2002;100:3203–8.
53. Schatteman GC, Dunnwald M, Jiao C. Biology of bone marrow-derived endothelial cell precursors. Am J Physiol Heart Circ Physiol 2007;292:H1–18.
54. Yoder MC, Mead LE, Prater D, et al. Redefining endothelial progenitor cells via clonal analysis and hematopoietic stem/progenitor cell principals. Blood 2007;109:1801–9.
55. Hamada H, Kim MK, Iwakura A, et al. Estrogen receptors alpha and beta mediate contribution of bone marrow-derived endothelial progenitor cells to functional recovery after myocardial infarction. Circulation 2006;114:2261–70.
56. Heil M, Ziegelhoeffer T, Mees B, et al. A different outlook on the role of bone marrow stem cells in vascular growth: bone marrow delivers software not hardware. Circ Res 2004;94:573–4.
57. Iwakura A, Shastry S, Luedemann C, et al. Estradiol enhances recovery after myocardial infarction by augmenting incorporation of bone marrow-derived endothelial progenitor cells into sites of ischemia-induced neovascularization via endothelial nitric oxide synthase-mediated activation of matrix metalloproteinase-9. Circulation 2006;113:1605–14.
58. Strehlow K, Werner N, Berweiler J, et al. Estrogen increases bone marrow-derived endothelial progenitor cell production and diminishes neointima formation. Circulation 2003;107:3059–65.
59. Dumont DJ, Fong GH, Puri MC, et al. Vascularization of the mouse embryo: a study of flk-1, tek, tie, and vascular endothelial growth factor expression during development. Dev Dyn 1995;203:80–92.
60. Nishikawa SI, Nishikawa S, Hirashima M, et al. Progressive lineage analysis by cell sorting and culture identifies FLK1+ve-cadherin+ cells at a diverging point of endothelial and hemopoietic lineages. Development 1998;125:1747–57.
61. Shalaby F, Rossant J, Yamaguchi TP, et al. Failure of blood-island formation and vasculogenesis in Flk-1-deficient mice. Nature 1995;376:62–6.
62. Vittet D, Prandini MH, Berthier R, et al. Embryonic stem cells differentiate in vitro to endothelial cells through successive maturation steps. Blood 1996;88:3424–31.
63. Aicher A, Zeiher AM, Dimmeler S. Mobilizing endothelial progenitor cells. Hypertension 2005;45:321–5.
64. Imanishi T, Hano T, Nishio I. Estrogen reduces endothelial progenitor cell senescence through augmentation of telomerase activity. J Hypertens 2005;23:1699–706.
65. Bolego C, Vegeto E, Pinna C, et al. Selective agonists of estrogen receptor isoforms: new perspectives for cardiovascular disease. Arterioscler Thromb Vasc Biol 2006;26:2192–9.

66. Gargett CE, Lederman FL, Lau TM, et al. Lack of correlation between vascular endothelial growth factor production and endothelial cell proliferation in the human endometrium. Hum Reprod 1999;14:2080–8.

67. Li XF, Gregory J, Ahmed A. Immunolocalisation of vascular endothelial growth factor in human endometrium. Growth Factors 1994;11:277–82.

68. Shifren JL, Tseng JF, Zaloudek CJ, et al. Ovarian steroid regulation of vascular endothelial growth factor in the human endometrium: implications for angiogenesis during the menstrual cycle and in the pathogenesis of endometriosis. J Clin Endocrinol Metab 1996;81:3112–8.

69. Heissig B, Hattori K, Dias S, et al. Recruitment of stem and progenitor cells from the bone marrow niche requires MMP-9 mediated release of kit-ligand. Cell 2002; 109:625–37.

70. Mints M, Jansson M, Sadeghi B, et al. Endometrial endothelial cells are derived from donor stem cells in a bone marrow transplant recipient. Hum Reprod 2008; 23:139–43.

71. Taylor HS. Endometrial cells derived from donor stem cells in bone marrow transplant recipients. JAMA 2004;292:81–5.

72. Jin DK, Shido K, Kopp HG, et al. Cytokine-mediated deployment of SDF-1 induces revascularization through recruitment of CXCR4+ hemangiocytes. Nat Med 2006;12:557–67.

73. Lapidot T, Dar A, Kollet O. How do stem cells find their way home? Blood 2005; 106:1901–10.

74. Sengenes C, Miranville A, Maumus M, et al. Chemotaxis and differentiation of human adipose tissue CD34+/CD31- progenitor cells: role of stromal derived factor-1 released by adipose tissue capillary endothelial cells. Stem Cells 2007; 25:2269–76.

75. Yamaguchi J, Kusano KF, Masuo O, et al. Stromal cell-derived factor-1 effects on ex vivo expanded endothelial progenitor cell recruitment for ischemic neovascularization. Circulation 2003;107:1322–8.

76. Elsheikh E, Sylven C, Ericzon BG, et al. Cyclic variability of stromal cell-derived factor-1 and endothelial progenitor cells during the menstrual cycle. Int J Mol Med 2011;27:221–6.

77. Matsubara K, Abe E, Matsubara Y, et al. Circulating endothelial progenitor cells during normal pregnancy and pre-eclampsia. Am J Reprod Immunol 2006;56: 79–85.

78. Freedman SB, Isner JM. Therapeutic angiogenesis for ischemic cardiovascular disease. J Mol Cell Cardiol 2001;33:379–93.

79. Isner JM. Still more debate over VEGF. Nat Med 2001;7:639–41.

80. Assmus B, Rolf A, Erbs S, et al. Clinical outcome 2 years after intracoronary administration of bone marrow-derived progenitor cells in acute myocardial infarction. Circ Heart Fail 2010;3:89–96.

81. Leistner DM, Schmitt J, Palm S, et al. Intracoronary administration of bone marrow-derived mononuclear cells and arrhythmic events in patients with chronic heart failure. Eur Heart J 2011;32:485–91.

82. Arbustini E, Dal B, Morbini P, et al. Plaque erosion is a major substrate for coronary thrombosis in acute myocardial infarction. Heart 1999;82(3):269–72.

# Imaging for Prevention

Leslee J. Shaw, PhD

**KEYWORDS**

- Imaging • Cardiovascular disease • Sudden cardiac death
- Coronary artery calcium

## CARDIOVASCULAR EPIDEMIOLOGY AND THE DETECTION GAP FOR IDENTIFYING HIGH-RISK INDIVIDUALS

Cardiovascular disease (CVD) deaths have declined considerably, with more than a 35% reduction during the past two decades, yet a sizable detection gap remains.[1] CVD remains the leading cause of morbidity and mortality in the United States and across the world, including in developing and developed nations for many decades.[2] Recent statistics in 2009 reveal that approximately 840,000 deaths were attributed to CVD, approximately 300,000 more deaths than reported for cancer.[3,4] Of those deaths, three-quarters were reported in previously asymptomatic individuals, raising the question as to whether screening for CVD is warranted in detecting potentially high-risk patients.

## WHAT IS IMAGING FOR PREVENTION?

With a sizable proportion of CVD events, including sudden cardiac death, occurring in previously asymptomatic, apparently healthy individuals, much discussion has occurred regarding whether screening beyond assessment of traditional cardiac risk factors (eg, diabetes and blood pressure) would improve detection of high-risk patients, who would benefit from more-intensive preventive therapies and lifestyle modifications.[1] The key to this approach is whether detection of high-risk patients would benefit from aggressive intervention, to the levels of secondary prevention, in terms of CVD risk reduction. The concept is that some asymptomatic patients may benefit from risk reduction with selective use of atherosclerosis imaging to identify high-risk individuals.

Several imaging and laboratory biomarkers have been proposed and undergone investigation during the past few decades. The current manuscript examines the concept of imaging for prevention, which largely includes tests that evaluate coronary and noncoronary arterial remodeling and plaque.[5] This article reviews the evidence of coronary artery calcium (CAC) as one measure of subclinical atherosclerosis in the major epicardial coronary arteries.[6,7]

Emory University School of Medicine, 1642 Clifton Road Northeast, Room 529, Atlanta, GA 30324, USA
E-mail address: lshaw3@emory.edu

Med Clin N Am 96 (2012) 103–112
doi:10.1016/j.mcna.2011.11.002
0025-7125/12/$ – see front matter © 2012 Elsevier Inc. All rights reserved.

## GLOBAL RISK SCORES

Accepted screening strategies include an office-based assessment integrating CVD risk factors into a global risk score, such as the Framingham risk score (FRS). The FRS is a risk prediction algorithm based on prognostic modeling derived and validated from the Framingham Heart Study based on risk factors, such as gender, age, diabetes, smoking history, blood pressure, and cholesterol measurements.[8] Based on the FRS, recommendations for prevention include reassurance and other public health recommendations for individuals with a low FRS, defined as a score of less than 10% coronary artery disease (CAD) death or myocardial infarction (MI) rate at 10 years.[9] Individuals with a low FRS encompass approximately 1 in 3 individuals. For individuals with low FRS, further risk assessment is recommended to be delayed for an additional 5 years with pharmacotherapy recommended only for those with identified abnormally elevated blood pressure or cholesterol values. A high FRS is defined in individuals with a 10-year CAD death or MI rate of greater than 20%. This category defines approximately 25% of adults and identifies individuals who are targeted for intensive therapeutic intervention and lifestyle modifications, with goals for management consistent with secondary prevention guidelines. Individuals with high FRS have CAD death and MI rates similar to those of patients with established CAD and are, therefore, called a risk equivalent cohort. Individuals with high FRS are not candidates for screening because their defined therapeutic intervention is clearly defined as consistent with secondary prevention goals.

The remaining 40% of individuals have a reported intermediate FRS with 10-year estimated CAD death or MI rates of 10% to 20%. This is the large population that is targeted for CVD screening. An American College of Cardiology Foundation (ACCF)/ American Heart Association (AHA) clinical practice guideline recently was published supporting the usefulness of screening in individuals with intermediate FRS.[10] The rationale for screening individuals with an intermediate FRS is that those with low-risk imaging findings would then be reclassified to a lower-risk group whereas those with high-risk findings would then be targeted for secondary prevention, similar to those with a high FRS (**Fig. 1**).

A challenge with the FRS is its limitations in accurately defining risk in sizable proportions of the population. In an earlier report, 70% of patients presenting with acute MI had a low FRS, with only 10% defined as high risk.[11] The FRS underestimates CVD risk in men less than 60 years of age and in women less than 70 years of age.[12] Key patient cohorts that are not defined in the FRS include individuals with a family history of CVD, those with an elevated high-sensitivity C-reactive protein greater than or equal to 3 mg/dL, or patients with the metabolic syndrome. A compelling cross-sectional study by Michos and colleagues,[13] of 2447 asymptomatic nondiabetic women, reported that 84% with significant CAC scores greater than or equal to the 75th percentile by age and gender were classified as low risk by the FRS.[13] The limitations of the FRS further support the usefulness of imaging as a means of more accurately detecting the pool of high-risk candidates for more-intensive prevention and targeted risk reduction strategies.

## SCREENING WITH CV IMAGING—CAN CT CAC SCORING IMPROVE DETECTION OF HIGH-RISK INDIVIDUALS?

Coronary calcification is a subcomponent of atheromatous plaque and can occur in the presymptomatic phase of the development of CAD.[6,7] The commonly applied CAC score was initially developed by Agatston and colleagues[14] and is easily calculated using the product of area of calcified plaque by the density of the plaque

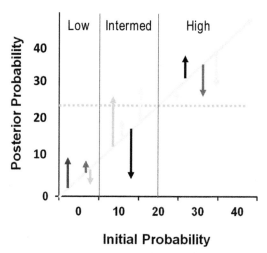

**Initial Probability**

**Fig. 1.** The goal of CVD screening is to target patients with an intermediate FRS. The rationale for targeting the intermediate FRS is that risk reclassification results in patients shifting to a low-risk or high-risk status. The likelihood of shifting to high-risk status for individuals with low FRS is small. The likelihood of shifting from a high FRS to low-risk status is small as well. Note the potential shift from the initial probability estimate to the posterior probability estimate.

(in Hounsfield units [HU]), where an HU from 130 to 199 is assigned a score of 1, 200 to 299 HU is assigned a score of 2, 300 to 399 HU is assigned a score of 3, and greater than 400 HU is assigned a score of 4. The CAC score is based on a linear scale with 5 prognostically distinct categories, including a score of 0 being no CAC, scores 1 to 99 mild CAC, scores 100 to 399 moderate CAC, scores 400 to 999 high-risk CAC, and scores greater than or equal to 1000 very high-risk CAC.

Abundant clinical and population registries have reported that CAC has established value in predicting cardiac events beyond the FRS.[10,15–18] This is vital information, particularly for those patients for whom the FRS results in notable limitations in accurate assessment of CAD risk. The prevalence of CAC varies by age, gender, and ethnicity.[19] In general, the prevalence of CAC correlates with the prevalence of obstructive coronary disease and is higher in men and older patients.[20]

There is a well-established relationship between CAC and major adverse cardiovascular (CV) events (MACE), with many reports of thousands of patients indicating a directly proportional relationship **(Fig. 2)**.[10,15–19] That is, the MACE rate increases with an increasing CAC score, with scores of 400 and higher having the highest event rate. From an ACCF expert consensus statement, a CAC score of 400 or higher was associated with an annual CAD death or MI rate of 2.0% or higher.[21,22] This threshold of 2.0% event rate is consistent with patients with known CAD and results in the distinction that a high-risk CAC score defines risk equivalent status at a level comparable to a patient with a prior diagnosis of CAD. Mortality associated with significant CAC scores of 100 or higher is decidedly higher in African American, Hispanic, and Asian patients compared with white individuals,[19] perhaps due to greater risk factor burden and comorbidity and reduced access to care and recommended guideline-accepted prevention practices.

Conversely, for individuals without CAC, an abundance of data indicates a very low MACE rate.[23] From a recent meta-analysis, the summary relative risk ratio was 0.15 (95% CI, 0.11–0.21) for no CAC compared with detectable CAC.[23] Min and

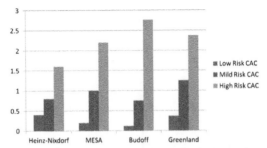

**Fig. 2.** Risk stratification with CAC scoring in 3 of the largest observational registries, including the Heinz Nixdorf Recall Study, the NIH-NHLBI–sponsored Multi-Ethnic Study of Atherosclerosis (MESA), and the Budoff registry. The data plot annual CVD death or MI rates for the Heinz Nixdorf and MESA registries with the Budoff series, showing all-cause mortality rates (per year).

colleagues[24] recently reported on significant factors contributing to conversion from no CAC to detectable CAC. Diabetes (hazard ratio 2.4), smoking (hazard ratio 1.8), and age greater than 40 years (hazard ratio 2.8) (all $P<.021$) were significant multivariable predictors of progression of a 0 CAC score to detectable calcified plaque.

Risk reclassification analyses have recently been touted as an important method of defining the added value of a given screening test (**Fig. 3**).[25] Using several analytic approaches, a simple reclassification index has been reported, indicating that when compared with the FRS, CAC subsequently reclassifies approximately two-thirds of individuals with intermediate FRS to low-risk status (ie, CAC $\leq$10), with nearly 1 in 10 patients with intermediate FRS identified as having a high-risk CAC score and reclassified to high-risk status.[17,26] Polonsky and colleagues[27] reported on the usefulness of the net reclassification index, based on data from the National Heart, Lung, and Blood Institute (NHLBI)-sponsored Multi-Ethnic Study of Atherosclerosis. In this report, Polonsky and colleagues[27] used 5-year risk estimates for incident coronary heart disease, using Cox regression modeling comparing the added classification of low-risk and high-risk status for CAC with the FRS alone. In this approach, the improved risk reclassification is compared, using a Cox model that includes age, gender, tobacco use, systolic blood pressure, antihypertensive medication, cholesterol measurements, and race/ethnicity compared with a second model that adds CAC to all of the variables included in the first model. The difference between these two models (ie, model 2 [risk factors + CAC] – model 1 [risk factors alone]) reveals

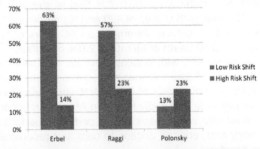

**Fig. 3.** Risk reclassification results that document a shift of a percentage of patients to low-risk and high-risk status after CAC scanning. The Erbel and Raggi series used simple reclassification analyses whereas the Polonsky series used the net reclassification improvement approach, which applies an increased rigor using Cox modeling.

any improvement in risk prediction. Based on this analysis, the net reclassification improvement was 0.25 (*P*<.001), or the CAC scan net reclassified 1 in 4 individuals. Specifically, the CAC scans risk reclassified an additional 23% of individuals with events as high risk and reclassified an additional 13% of individuals without events as low risk compared with the FRS.

Based on a recent compilation of evidence in the ACCF/AHA clinical practice guideline on detection of high-risk asymptomatic individuals, the following recommendations for use of CAC have been published[10]:

1. Class IIa recommendation—it is reasonable to perform a CAC scan for CV risk assessment in asymptomatic adults at intermediate FRS.[10]
2. Class IIb recommendation—it may be reasonable to perform a CAC scan for CV risk assessment persons at low to intermediate FRS.[10]
3. Class III recommendation—a CAC scan should not be performed in individuals with a low FRS for CV risk assessment purposes due to the low event rate in this population.[10]

Although the evidence on effective risk stratification and risk reclassification has been reported with CAC, the evidence on targeted therapeutic intervention guided by CAC scoring is minimal.[28] Several trials have reported on the usefulness of statin therapy to slow CAC progression. A recent meta-analysis reported no benefit with the use of statins to reduce CAC progression in 2051 enrolled patients (summary *P* = 0.40). From the Prospective Army Coronary Calcium Project (PACC), a total of 450 asymptomatic US Army (39–45 y, 79% male) personnel were enrolled in a randomized trial.[29] In this trial, individuals were randomized to receive a CAC score or to be managed based on their FRS alone, with the primary endpoint a change in the FRS. This trial evaluated whether knowledge of a patient's CAC score resulted in improved preventive care such that a reduced FRS would be observed. At 1 year, the mean absolute risk change in the FRS was +0.30 for those who received CAC results and +0.36 for those with the FRS alone (*P* = .81). These negative trial results were in controvert to prior findings of improved adherence to statin therapy for those patients with evidence of CAC.[30] Some investigators have criticized the PACC trial as largely enrolling younger individuals who may not reflect the general population with more prevalent risk factors and CAC. More recently, the Early Identification of Subclinical Atherosclerosis by Noninvasive Imaging Research (EISNER) trial results were reported.[31,32] This trial was similar to the PACC trial in that it randomized patients to a CAC scan versus no CAC scan using a 2:1 randomization scheme (675 individuals in the no-scan group and 1372 in the scan group). The main trial results revealed a 0.7% 4-year increase in the FRS in the no-scan group compared with a 0.002% increase in the FRS for those in the CAC scan group (*P* = .003). Compared with the no-scan arm, individuals undergoing CAC scanning exhibited favorable improvements in systolic blood pressure (*P* = .02), low-density lipoprotein cholesterol (*P* = .04), waist circumference, and weight loss for overweight and obese enrollees (*P* = .01 and *P* = .07, respectively).

This evidence from the EISNER trial provides substantial evidence that use of the CAC scan resulted in changes in patient management and preventive care. These data represent a significant advancement in the body of evidence for CAC scanning. A larger trial of the effectiveness of the FRS with CAC scanning compared with the FRS alone for improvement in MACE at 5 years is currently being evaluated at the National Institutes of Health (NIH)-NHLBI.

One additional consideration is what additional testing should patients with high-risk CAC findings undergo for assessment of inducible ischemia (**Fig. 4**). There are also

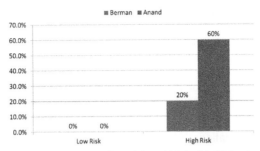

**Fig. 4.** Incidence of inducible ischemia in low-risk and high-risk CAC scores from 2 series. The Berman series reports the incidence of ischemia encompassing 5% or more of the myocardium, whereas the Anand series is in type 2 diabetics in whom the frequency of ischemia is decidedly higher.

several observational series reporting on the usefulness of follow-up stress myocardial perfusion imaging for those patients with a high-risk CAC score of 400 or higher.[23,32,33] Approximately 10% and 20% of patients with CAC scores of 400 to 999 and greater than 1000 have moderate-severe ischemia.[33] In a series of 510 type 2 diabetics, the prevalence of ischemia approached 50% for those with a CAC of 400 or higher.[34] It seems reasonable, therefore, to consider follow-up stress testing with the goal of initiating anti-ischemic therapy in patients with inducible ischemia. Coronary angiography may be considered for those with moderate-severe ischemia. Although the use of coronary revascularization in asymptomatic patients is controversial, the assessment of the extent and severity of obstructive CAD may be reasonable given the risk associated with moderate-severe ischemia combined with a high-risk CAC score.

## CAC SCREENING—THE BENEFIT OUTWEIGHS THE PROJECTED RISK

As discussed previously, there is substantial evidence that imaging with CAC scanning can be used to improve preventive care. CAC scanning can result in (1) early detection of subclinical atherosclerosis, (2) improved identification of high-risk individuals who are in need of targeted secondary preventive care, and (3) guiding management decisions, including assessing the burden of silent ischemia.

The EISNER trial also examined the cost implications of CAC scanning by reporting on downstream CAD testing patterns.[31,32] Many of the arguments against screening for CVD have been that initial screening will result in an onslaught of downstream resource consumption. From the EISNER trial, downstream diagnostic testing with stress testing (echocardiography or nuclear imaging) occurred largely in patients with high CAC scores of 400 or higher.[32] Approximately one-third of patients with a high-risk CAC score greater than 400 underwent stress echocardiography or nuclear imaging within 1 year of testing. By comparison, for those with a CAC score of 0 to 10, only 0.3% underwent coronary angiography. Thus, the majority of downstream resource consumption was limited to patients with significant CAC scores, generally those of 100 or higher. Average costs for testing were approximately $30 for CAC scores less than 100 but increased proportionally for higher scores, ranging from $145 to $1438 for scores from 100 to greater than or equal to 1000. From the main trial results, individuals with a 0 CAC score had lower costs when compared to patients randomized to the no scan arm ($P = .001$). These included fewer downstream procedures ($P = .001$) and reduced costs for statins ($P = .024$), aspirin ($P = .016$), and diabetic ($P = .024$) medications.[31] Thus, it seems that the benefit of CAC scanning supports the economic burden of testing in that CAC scanning does not seem to induce excessive testing and downstream CAC procedure use is limited to those with high-risk findings on CAC imaging.

One final consideration is that CAC scanning is associated with patient exposure to ionizing radiation.[35,36] There are several caveats for readers to understand, including the principle that exposure to ionizing radiation should be limited to patients for whom the clinical need and information gained is substantial (in this case, those with an intermediate FRS [discussed previously]). Thus, exposure and referral to any tests with associated ionizing radiation should be limited to patients for whom a sizable improvement in knowledge may be gained. The evidence with CAC does support substantial improvement in risk detection and targeted preventive therapeutic management. Recent guidelines support CAC screening in individuals with an intermediate FRS, for whom risk reclassification is greatest. Thus, this discussion of application of CAC scanning is limited to those patients with an intermediate FRS. Another factor is that there is no direct evidence that exposure of a given patient to ionizing radiation from a medical procedure has been directly linked to cancer. There is a projected cancer risk, however, that is based on higher exposures in individuals exposed to high doses ($\geq$100 mSv), from observations of related cancer incidence after World War II bombings in Hiroshima and Nagasaki. The extrapolation of a high-dose exposure ($\geq$100 mSv) to low-dose exposure (as is required for most medical procedures) is controversial and is associated with uncertainty around the projected cancer risk estimates. Thus, the medical community applies a cautionary note of limiting exposure to those individuals who benefit greatly from imaging.

The average effective dose of ionizing radiation for CAC scanning is 2 mSv, substantially lower than that for other CT or single-photon emission CT (SPECT) imaging procedures.[35,37–39] Projected cancer risk estimates have been calculated and report that for a base case of a 60-year-old patient, exposure with CAC scanning results in an additional 2.5 and 1 incident cancer cases for every 10,000 patients screened.[36] This is compared with 9 to 17 incident cancer cases projected for every 10,000 patients scanned with coronary CT angiography or myocardial perfusion SPECT as a result of higher effective doses, in the range of 8 to 15 mSv. The exposure and projected cancer risk, therefore, are low and recommendations of CAC use are solely for those with an intermediate FRS would limit use to those who truly benefit from testing.

## SUMMARY

The evidence with CAC scanning is impressive and shows effective risk stratification of patients with low-risk to very high-risk findings. Moreover, CAC scanning can provide a necessary link to improve patient compliance and focus preventive care, resulting in an improved FRS. Although no comparative effectiveness data are available, in particular comparing CAC scanning to a test without ionizing radiation, current evidence supports the clinical benefit of testing that far exceeds the small projected cancer risk. Finally, it seems that the economic burden of CAC scanning is limited to those patients in need of additional testing (ie, those with a high-risk scan) and does not induce unwarranted testing. These data in synthesis provide tremendous evidence of a highly effective, efficient, and safe procedure to be applied as an imaging procedure for guiding primary and secondary prevention strategies.

## REFERENCES

1. Pasternak RC, Abrams J, Greenland P, et al. 34th Bethesda conference: task force #1—identification of coronary heart disease risk: is there a detection gap? J Am Coll Cardiol 2003;41:1863–74.

2. Vitola JV, Shaw LJ, Allam AH, et al. Assessing the need for nuclear cardiology and other advanced cardiac imaging modalities in the developing world. J Nucl Cardiol 2009;16:956–61.

3. Lloyd-Jones D, Adams R, Carnethon M, et al. Heart disease and stroke statistics—2009 update: a report from the American heart association statistics committee and stroke statistics subcommittee. Circulation 2009;119:e21–181.

4. Roger VL, Go AS, Lloyd-Jones DM, et al. Heart disease and stroke statistics—2011 update: a report from the American heart association. Circulation 2011; 123:e18–209.

5. Shaw LJ, Berman DS, Blumenthal RS, et al. Clinical imaging for prevention: directed strategies for improved detection of presymptomatic patients with undetected atherosclerosis—part I: clinical imaging for prevention. J Nucl Cardiol 2008;15:e6–19.

6. O'Rourke RA, Brundage BH, Froelicher VF, et al. American college of cardiology/American heart association expert consensus document on electron-beam computed tomography for the diagnosis and prognosis of coronary artery disease. J Am Coll Cardiol 2000;36:326–40.

7. O'Rourke RA, Brundage BH, Froelicher VF, et al. American College of Cardiology/American Heart Association Expert Consensus document on electron-beam computed tomography for the diagnosis and prognosis of coronary artery disease. Circulation 2000;102:126–40.

8. Wilson PW, D'Agostino RB, Levy D, et al. Prediction of coronary heart disease using risk factor categories. Circulation 1998;97:1837–47.

9. Greenland P, Smith SC Jr, Grundy SM. Improving coronary heart disease risk assessment in asymptomatic people: role of traditional risk factors and noninvasive cardiovascular tests. Circulation 2001;104:1863–7.

10. Greenland P, Alpert JS, Beller GA, et al. 2010 ACCF/AHA guideline for assessment of cardiovascular risk in asymptomatic adults: a report of the American college of cardiology foundation/American heart association task force on practice guidelines. J Am Coll Cardiol 2010;56:e50–103.

11. Akosah KO, Schaper A, Cogbill C, et al. Preventing myocardial infarction in the young adult in the first place: how do the National Cholesterol Education Panel III guidelines perform? J Am Coll Cardiol 2003;41:1475–9.

12. Nasir K, Michos ED, Blumenthal RS, et al. Detection of high-risk young adults and women by coronary calcium and National Cholesterol Education Program Panel III guidelines. J Am Coll Cardiol 2005;46:1931–6.

13. Michos ED, Nasir K, Braunstein JB, et al. Framingham risk equation underestimates subclinical atherosclerosis risk in asymptomatic women. Atherosclerosis 2006;184:201–6.

14. Agatston AS, Janowitz WR, Hildner FJ, et al. Quantification of coronary artery calcium using ultrafast computed tomography. J Am Coll Cardiol 1990;15:827–32.

15. Detrano R, Guerci AD, Carr JJ, et al. Coronary calcium as a predictor of coronary events in four racial or ethnic groups. N Engl J Med 2008;358:1336–45.

16. Budoff MJ, Shaw LJ, Liu ST, et al. Long-term prognosis associated with coronary calcification: observations from a registry of 25,253 patients. J Am Coll Cardiol 2007;49:1860–70.

17. Raggi P, Gongora MC, Gopal A, et al. Coronary artery calcium to predict all-cause mortality in elderly men and women. J Am Coll Cardiol 2008;52:17–23.

18. Raggi P, Shaw LJ, Berman DS, et al. Prognostic value of coronary artery calcium screening in subjects with and without diabetes. J Am Coll Cardiol 2004;43:1663–9.

19. Nasir K, Shaw LJ, Liu ST, et al. Ethnic differences in the prognostic value of coronary artery calcification for all-cause mortality. J Am Coll Cardiol 2007;50:953–60.
20. Nasir K, Raggi P, Rumberger JA, et al. Coronary artery calcium volume scores on electron beam tomography in 12,936 asymptomatic adults. Am J Cardiol 2004; 93:1146–9.
21. Greenland P, Bonow RO, Brundage BH, et al. ACCF/AHA 2007 clinical expert consensus document on coronary artery calcium scoring by computed tomography in global cardiovascular risk assessment and in evaluation of patients with chest pain: a report of the American College of Cardiology Foundation Clinical Expert Consensus Task Force (ACCF/AHA Writing Committee to Update the 2000 Expert Consensus Document on Electron Beam Computed Tomography) developed in collaboration with the Society of Atherosclerosis Imaging and Prevention and the Society of Cardiovascular Computed Tomography. J Am Coll Cardiol 2007;49:378–402.
22. Greenland P, Bonow RO, Brundage BH, et al. ACCF/AHA 2007 clinical expert consensus document on coronary artery calcium scoring by computed tomography in global cardiovascular risk assessment and in evaluation of patients with chest pain: a report of the American College of Cardiology Foundation Clinical Expert Consensus Task Force (ACCF/AHA Writing Committee to Update the 2000 Expert Consensus Document on Electron Beam Computed Tomography). Circulation 2007;115:402–26.
23. Sarwar A, Shaw LJ, Shapiro MD, et al. Diagnostic and prognostic value of absence of coronary artery calcification. JACC Cardiovasc Imaging 2009;2: 675–88.
24. Min JK, Lin FY, Gidseg DS, et al. Determinants of coronary calcium conversion among patients with a normal coronary calcium scan: what is the "warranty period" for remaining normal? J Am Coll Cardiol 2010;55:1110–7.
25. Shaw LJ. The new era of risk reclassification in cardiovascular imaging. J Nucl Cardiol 2011;18:536–7.
26. Erbel R, Mohlenkamp S, Moebus S, et al. Coronary risk stratification, discrimination, and reclassification improvement based on quantification of subclinical coronary atherosclerosis: the Heinz Nixdorf Recall Study. J Am Coll Cardiol 2010;56:1397–406.
27. Polonsky TS, McClelland RL, Jorgensen NW, et al. Coronary artery calcium score and risk classification for coronary heart disease prediction. JAMA 2010;303: 1610–6.
28. Oudkerk M, Stillman AE, Halliburton SS, et al. Coronary artery calcium screening: current status and recommendations from the European Society of Cardiac Radiology and North American Society for Cardiovascular Imaging. Eur Radiol 2008; 18:2785–807.
29. O'Malley PG, Feuerstein IM, Taylor AJ. Impact of electron beam tomography, with or without case management, on motivation, behavioral change, and cardiovascular risk profile: a randomized controlled trial. JAMA 2003;289: 2215–23.
30. Kalia NK, Miller LG, Nasir K, et al. Visualizing coronary calcium is associated with improvements in adherence to statin therapy. Atherosclerosis 2006;185: 394–9.
31. Rozanski A, Gransar H, Shaw LJ, et al. Impact of coronary artery calcium scanning on coronary risk factors and downstream testing the EISNER (Early Identification of Subclinical Atherosclerosis by Noninvasive Imaging Research) prospective randomized trial. J Am Coll Cardiol 2011;57:1622–32.

32. Shaw LJ, Min JK, Budoff M, et al. Induced cardiovascular procedural costs and resource consumption patterns after coronary artery calcium screening: results from the EISNER (Early Identification of Subclinical Atherosclerosis by Noninvasive Imaging Research) study. J Am Coll Cardiol 2009;54:1258–67.

33. Berman DS, Wong ND, Gransar H, et al. Relationship between stress-induced myocardial ischemia and atherosclerosis measured by coronary calcium tomography. J Am Coll Cardiol 2004;44:923–30.

34. Anand DV, Lim E, Hopkins D, et al. Risk stratification in uncomplicated type 2 diabetes: prospective evaluation of the combined use of coronary artery calcium imaging and selective myocardial perfusion scintigraphy. Eur Heart J 2006;27: 713–21.

35. Kim KP, Einstein AJ, Berrington de Gonzalez A. Coronary artery calcification screening: estimated radiation dose and cancer risk. Arch Intern Med 2009; 169:1188–94.

36. Berrington de Gonzalez A, Mahesh M, Kim KP, et al. Projected cancer risks from computed tomographic scans performed in the united states in 2007. Arch Intern Med 2009;169:2071–7.

37. Geleijns J, Joemai RM, Dewey M, et al. Radiation exposure to patients in a multi-center coronary angiography trial (core 64). AJR Am J Roentgenol 2011;196: 1126–32.

38. Halliburton SS, Abbara S, Chen MY, et al. SCCT guidelines on radiation dose and dose-optimization strategies in cardiovascular CT. J Cardiovasc Comput Tomogr 2011;5:198–224.

39. Einstein AJ. Radiation risk from cardiac ct and nuclear cardiology: addressing concerns with innovative solutions. J Nucl Cardiol 2011;18:561.

# Genomics: Is It Ready for Primetime?

Sonny Dandona, MD, FRCPC[a],
Alexandre F.R. Stewart, BSch, MSc, PhD[b],
Robert Roberts, MD, FRCPC, MACC[c],*

KEYWORDS

- Coronary artery disease • Genomics
- Single nucleotide polymorphism • Sequence variation

Coronary artery disease (CAD) is the leading killer in the industrialized world.[1] Its presentation is varied, from gradual narrowing of the major epicardial conduits that leads to the clinical syndrome of angina to plaque rupture and overlying thrombosis that leads to its most feared consequence, that of sudden and unexpected death in the young. It has long been understood that although there are several modifiable risk factors that are involved in its pathogenesis, there is a hereditary component that strongly affects the risk of disease. Elucidation of the sequence variation that underlies heredity is essential to the more comprehensive identification of those at risk and to provide novel therapeutic targets.

The completion of the Human Genome Project demonstrated that coding sequences occupied no more than 2% of the genome.[2] Intervening intronic sequences account for a further 8% to 10% of the genome. It was perhaps reasonably concluded that up to 90% of the genome was not essential and, therefore, referred to as junk DNA.[2] It became apparent, however, that a large proportion of the so-called junk DNA was indeed transcribed and that several classes of regulatory RNAs exist.[3] These classes are not protein encoding but function to regulate the expression of coding mRNA. There exist at least 3 categories of regulatory RNAs, namely the micro RNAs, the intermediate RNAs, and the long noncoding RNAs.[4] The exact roles of these RNAs are being elucidated, but it is apparent that the micro RNAs exert their action by reducing the number of mRNA transcripts that are ultimately transcribed either by binding to the 3-prime end of the mRNA and preventing its translation or promoting its degradation.[4]

[a] Faculty of Medicine, McGill University, McIntyre Medical Building, 3655 promenade Sir William Osler Montreal, Quebec H3G 1Y6, Canada
[b] Ruddy Canadian Cardiovascular Genetics Centre, 40 Ruskin Street, Ottawa, Ontario K2Y 4W7, Canada
[c] Ruddy Canadian Cardiovascular Genetics Centre, University of Ottawa Heart Institute, 40 Ruskin Street, H-2404A, Ottawa, Ontario K2Y 4W7, Canada
* Corresponding author.
E-mail address: rroberts@ottawaheart.ca

Med Clin N Am 96 (2012) 113–122
doi:10.1016/j.mcna.2012.01.018
0025-7125/12/$ – see front matter © 2012 Elsevier Inc. All rights reserved.

medical.theclinics.com

## DNA SEQUENCE VARIATION AND THE HapMap PROJECT

It has been recently described that 98.5% of the genome is invariant between individuals. The logical extension is that heredity is determined by genetic variation present in the remaining 1.5% of the genome. This variation takes 2 forms: DNA sequence variation characterized by a single base substitution at a given locus, a single nucleotide polymorphism (SNP) and variation in the number of copies of large segments of DNA sequence, referred to as copy number variants. SNPs are responsible for 80% of genetic variation causing differences in the phenotype such as hair color, height and predisposition to disease.[5] Each genome harbors approximately 3 million SNPs. The HapMap project annotated these SNPs with respect to their location within the genome.[6] The HapMap project provided the DNA markers for the development of the gene chips that in turn facilitated the execution of genome-wide association studies (GWAS) that probed the genetic underpinnings of complex genetic disease.[7]

## MONOGENIC DISORDERS

Thus far, genetic investigation has centered on identifying those variants that were responsible for the development of monogenic disorders, conditions whereby the genetic lesion is both necessary and sufficient for the development of the phenotype of interest. Considerable progress has been made in delineating the genetic basis for these conditions. These bases include familial hypercholesterolemia,[8] congenital long QT syndrome,[9] hypertrophic cardiomyopathy,[10] and Wolff-Parkinson-White syndrome.[11] Methodologically, kindreds of at least 2 generations are identified that contain both affected and nonaffected members. Linkage analysis is then performed with a few hundred DNA markers whereby the approximate location of the gene of interest is identified if a given marker segregates with the phenotype of interest in a frequency greater than that expected by mere chance.[11] There are approximately 6000 disorders that seem to be monogenic of which 2000 have been mapped.

## GENETIC UNDERPINNINGS OF COMMON COMPLEX DISEASES AND THE GWAS

The genetics that underlie complex disease is quite different in that multiple loci of modest biologic importance act in concert to modulate the likelihood of developing disease. The identification of these loci is not amenable to the type of linkage analysis that is used in monogenic disorders; the use of several hundred markers in the genome lacks the necessary resolution to identify these variants.[7]

The development of the microarray that interrogated several hundred thousand SNPs permitted the investigation of complex genetic disease in a case-control format. That is, SNP frequency is compared in individuals with the phenotype of interest to that in appropriate controls. If the frequency of a SNP is greater in patients than controls it is said to be risk conferring. Conversely, if the frequency is lower among patients, it is said to be protective.

## 9p21: THE FIRST AND MOST ROBUST GENETIC RISK FACTOR TO EMERGE FROM GWAS

The first series of GWAS led to the striking observation that there exists sequence variation at chromosome 9p21 that is present in 75% of the population (25% of the population is homozygous for the variant, whereas a further 50% are heterozygous) that confers a risk for CAD/myocardial infarction (MI).[12–14] Homozygosity confers a twofold risk for the development of MI. Although the first descriptions of the CAD association were in Caucasian populations,[12–14] the association has since been described in

Chinese,[15] Korean,[16] Japanese,[16] and South Asian populations.[17] However, 9p21 does not seem to impart risk for CAD in African Americans.[18]

Interestingly, the variant has also been shown to associate with the development of both abdominal aortic aneurysm and intracranial aneurysm.[19] This finding raises the possibility that 9p21 promotes defects in the vessel wall that promote both aneurysm formation in the vessel and atherogenesis. There are data that suggest gene dosage of the variant correlates with disease severity; in a cohort with established CAD, although heterozygosity significantly increased the likelihood of development of 3 vessel disease when compared with noncarriers, homozygosity further significantly increased this likelihood. Of note, once controlled for disease severity, 9p21 did not seem to influence the likelihood of MI.[20] Consistent with this observation, a recent study demonstrated that in a cohort of patients with established disease, although gene dosage of 9p21 was not predictive of MI, it was predictive of subsequent revascularization.[21]

The elucidation of the mechanism by which 9p21 exerts its action on the vasculature has been complicated by the fact the sequence variants lie in a so-called gene desert, the nearest annotated genes, cyclin-dependent kinase N2A (CDKN2A) and cyclin-dependent kinase N2B (CDKN2B) lie 100,000 base pairs away from the lead SNP, rs1333049. Moreover, 9p21 does not seem to exert its effect via the known modifiable risk factors.[12]

CDKN2A and CDKN2B are cell cycle inhibitors that act on both p53 and retinoblastoma protein pathways. Jarinova and colleagues[22] reported a reduced expression of CDKN2B in association with the risk genotype in individuals without disease. Recently Visel and colleagues[23] deleted a 70-kilobase (kb) region from chromosome 4 in a mouse, a region that is analogous to that of the 58-kb region on 9p21 in humans. Following deletion, decreased expression of both CDKN2A and CDKN2B was noted with a corresponding increase in smooth muscle cell proliferation. However, increased atheromatosis was not noted in the aortas in the mice with a deleted 70-kb region. It could be argued that deletion of the region does not appropriately model 9p21 sequence variation. Furthermore, there exists only modest homology between the mouse and human 9p21 locus that potentially compromises its ability to reliably model 9p21 sequence variation in the human.

The 9p21 is particularly rich in enhancers.[24] The lead SNP, rs10757278, lies in the enhancer ECAD9 and interferes with the binding of the transcription factor STAT1.[24] STAT 1 modulates inflammation and expression of interferons and, therefore, may provide a link between inflammation and the pathogenesis of CAD.[24] Importantly, it may validate this as an approach to identify regulatory elements in noncoding regions that have been described by GWAS.

## AN ABUNDANCE OF GENETIC RISK VARIANTS DISCOVERED BY GWAS

The association of 9p21 with CAD was described in the spring of 2007. Since then, there have been a series of publications that have described the association of various DNA sequence variants with CAD or one of its related phenotypes (**Table 1**).[14,17,25–29] It was immediately clear that these variants impart a risk that is modest at best (relative risk 1.1–1.25) and that their identification would require the enrollment of tens of thousands of cases and a similar number of controls. Thus, a consortium was formed from 12 GWAS that investigated CAD. CARDIoGRAM (Coronary Artery Disease Genome-wide Replication and Meta Analysis) included 86,995 individuals (22,233 patients vs 64,762 controls) of European ancestry in its discovery set, each of whom was genotyped using 1 million SNP arrays. SNPs that demonstrated a consistent trend across

**Table 1**
Genetic variants associated with CAD discovered by GWAS and replicated in independent populations

| Chromosome | SNP | Nearby Genes | Risk Allele Frequency (Allele) | Odds Ratio (95% CI) |
|---|---|---|---|---|
| 1p32.3 | rs11206510 | PCSK9 | 0.82 (T) | 1.15 (1.10–1.21) |
| 1p13.3 | rs599839 | SORT1 | 0.78 (A) | 1.29 (1.18–1.40) |
| 1q41 | rs17465637 | MIA3 | 0.74 (C) | 1.20 (1.12–1.30) |
| 2q33.1 | rs6725887 | WDR12 | 0.15 (C) | 1.16 (1.10–1.22) |
| 3q22.3 | rs2306374 | MRAS | 0.18 (C) | 1.15 (1.11–1.19) |
| 6p24.1 | rs12526453 | PHACTR1 | 0.67 (C) | 1.13 (1.09–1.17) |
| 6q25.3 | rs3798220 | LPA | 0.02 (C) | 1.92 (1.48–2.49) |
| 9p21.3 | rs4977574 | CDKN2A,CDKN2B | 0.46 (G) | 1.25 (1.18–1.31) |
| 10q11.21 | rs1746048 | CXCL12 | 0.87 (C) | 1.33 (1.20–1.48) |
| 12q24.12 | rs3184504 | SH2B3 | 0.44 (T) | 1.13 (1.08–1.18) |
| 19p13.2 | rs1122608 | LDLR | 0.77 (G) | 1.14 (1.09–1.19) |
| 21q22.11 | rs9982601 | MRPS6 | 0.15 (T) | 1.19 (1.13–1.27) |
| 1p32.2 | rs17114036 | PPAP2B | 0.91 (A) | 1.17 (1.13–1.22) |
| 6p21.31 | rs17609940 | ANKS1A | 0.75 (G) | 1.07 (1.05–1.10) |
| 6q23.2 | rs12190287 | TCF21 | 0.62 (C) | 1.08 (1.06–1.10) |
| 7q32.2 | rs11556924 | ZC3HC1 | 0.62 (C) | 1.09 (1.07–1.12) |
| 9q34.2 | rs579459 | ABO | 0.21 (C) | 1.10 (1.07–1.13) |
| 10q24.32 | rs12413409 | CYP17A1, CNNM2, NT5C2 | 0.89 (G) | 1.12 (1.08–1.16) |
| 11q23.3 | rs964184 | ZNF259, APOA5-A4-C3-A1 | 0.13 (G) | 1.13 (1.10–1.16) |
| 13q34 | rs4773144 | COL4A1, COL4A2 | 0.44 (G) | 1.07 (1.05–1.09) |
| 14q32.2 | rs2895811 | HHIPL1 | 0.43 (C) | 1.07 (1.05–1.10) |
| 17p13.3 | rs216172 | SMG6, SRR | 0.37 (C) | 1.07 (1.05–1.09) |
| 17p11.2 | rs12936587 | RASD1, SMCR3, PEMT | 0.56 (G) | 1.07 (1.05–1.09) |
| 17q21.32 | rs46522 | UBE2Z, GIP, ATP5G1, SNF8 | 0.53 (T) | 1.06 (1.04–1.08) |
| 10q23.31 | rs1412444 | LIPA | 0.34 (T) | 1.09 (1.07–1.12) |
| 11q22.3 | rs974819 | PDGF | 0.29 (T) | 1.07 (1.04–1.09) |
| 7q22.3 | rs10953541 | BCAP29 | 0.75 (C) | 1.08 (1.05–1.11) |
| 10p11.23 | rs2505083 | KIAA1462 | 0.42 (C) | 1.07 (1.04–1.09) |
| 6p24.1 | rs6903956 | C6orf105 | 0.07 (A) | 1.65 (1.44–1.90) |
| 15q25.1 | rs1994016 | ADAMTS7 | 0.60 (C) | 1.19 (1.13–1.24) |

Abbreviation: CI, confidence interval.

studies and achieved genome-wide significance on meta-analysis ($5.0 \times 10\text{-}8$) were carried through to a second replication phase in a sample size of 56,682.[30] This process led to the discovery of 13 new variants and confirmation of 10 previously described variants.[28]

The Coronary Artery Disease (C4D) Consortium discovered a further 5 loci in a combined sample comprised of Caucasians and South Asians. There did not seem to exist race-specific association.[17]

Using similar methodology, Reilly and colleagues[31] confirmed the association of ADAMTS7, previously described by C4D with coronary atherosclerosis. However, they refined the observation by demonstrating that ADAMTS7 did not associate with MI. Furthermore, they described the association of the ABO locus with MI in the presence of coronary atherosclerosis.[31] It is postulated that the genes for A and B impart a risk for MI by adding a carbohydrate moiety to von Willebrand factor, thereby lengthening its half-life with an associated risk for thrombosis.[31]

Wang and colleagues[29] described the association of a new locus with CAD following a 3-stage GWAS that seems, thus far, to exert its action only in the Chinese Han population. Thus, a total of 30 genetic variants has been discovered and replicated in large sample sizes as indicated in **Table 1**.

## MECHANISMS UNDERLYING SNP ASSOCIATION DISCOVERED IN GWAS

Of the loci discovered by GWAS, only 6 seem to operate via known risk factors. This finding would suggest that most exert their action via pathways that are hitherto unknown. Therefore, as these pathways are unraveled, so too will novel targets for intervention.

1p13 was identified in the Wellcome Trust Case Control Consortium[14] and found to have a strong association with plasma low-density lipoprotein (LDL). Through a series of experiments, it was shown that 1p13 creates a C/enhancer-binding protein (CCAAT/EBP) transcription factor–binding site and, thereby, alters the expression of the SORT1, which in turn modulates plasma LDL and very low-density lipoprotein (VLDL) levels by altering hepatic VLDL secretion.[32] This finding demonstrates the ability of noncoding SNPs discovered via GWAS to directly modify commonly measured clinical indices.

## PHARMACOGENOMICS

DNA sequence variation can affect the response to medical pharmacotherapy. This sequence variation usually exists in proteins that affect drug metabolism and, therefore, modulate pharmacodynamic and pharmacokinetic profiles.

Recently a series of articles that focused on polymorphisms in cytochrome P450 isoforms that are involved in the metabolism of the thienopyridines, clopidogrel and prasugrel, identified an SNP in the gene-encoding cytochrome P450 2C19 whose carriage tripled the risk of stent thrombosis in those patients who were administered clopidogrel.[33] This finding was not the case in the population in whom prasugrel was administered.[34] It is evident that elucidation of the genotype could potentially be advantageous in determining which patients could benefit from the administration of prasugrel over clopidogrel.

Coumadin is the cornerstone drug in stroke prophylaxis in the context of atrial fibrillation. It is also used in the treatment of venous thromboembolic disease and is administered following the placement of prosthetic metallic valves. Until recently, titration of warfarin dosage was undertaken blindly. Recent studies have demonstrated that mutations in cytochrome P450 2C9 and the target of warfarin, vitamin K epoxide reductase complex subunit 1 (VKORC1), reduce the time to achieve therapeutic international normalized ratios (INRs) and supratherapeutic INRs.[35] A subsequent study compared blinded prescription of warfarin with genotype-guided prescription; at 6 months, hospitalizations for hemorrhage were 28% less frequent in the group in whom prescription was guided.[36]

Genomics can also be used to identify mutations that predispose to drug complications. Statin-induced myopathy is a complication of hydroxy-methylglutaryl (HMG) coenzyme A inhibitors. A mutation in the ion transporter SLCO1B1 was identified by GWAS and shown to confer a 17-fold risk for the development of this sequel in homozygotes.[37]

A more comprehensive inventory of such SNPs will facilitate a transition to a more personalized approach to health care.

## INFORMATION GLEANED FROM CAD GENETIC RISK VARIANTS

In less than 5 years, 30 genetic risk variants have been identified and replicated in large, independent populations. Based on these 30 variants, the following information will be insightful for future studies:

1. Only 6 of the risk variants mediate their effect through known risk factors for CAD. This observation indicates several mechanisms contributing to the pathogenesis of CAD are yet to be elucidated.
2. The number of risk variants for CAD per individual varies from 15 to 37.
3. The top 10th percentile versus the lowest 10th percentile is associated with an odds ratio for CAD of 1.88 and 0.55 respectively.
4. The relative risk of each variant for CAD varies from 6% to 17%.
5. Most genetic variants are associated with higher risk for early onset than for late-onset CAD.
6. Of the genetic risk variants for CAD, more than 70% are located in DNA sequences that do not code for protein. This finding would imply that most of these polymorphisms exert their effect through regulation of protein coding sequences.
7. These variants indicate several potential targets for the development of novel therapy that are probably a requisite for comprehensive prevention and treatment of CAD.

## ADVANTAGES OF DNA RISK VARIANTS OVER CONVENTIONAL BIOMARKERS

In contrast to a biomarker, such as cholesterol, sampling for DNA only needs to be performed once in a lifetime. The DNA risk variant does not change in one's lifetime. Furthermore, DNA variants do not vary with meals, drugs, or gender, thus, a single blood test can be performed at birth without the necessity for ever repeating the blood test. Furthermore, a single DNA risk variant may have multiple effects.

## ROLE OF GENETIC RISK VARIANTS IN PREDICTION AND TREATMENT OF CORONARY ARTERY DISEASE

Genetic risk variants add 2 potential benefits, namely, early prediction of disease to provide more effective prevention and as new targets for more effective and comprehensive treatment. Are the genetic risk variants ready for primetime? The current answer to this question is no. However, it is probably not because their risk is not significant but because it is premature in terms of altering management. For example, 9p21 is a predictor of the severity of CAD as reflected by the number of coronary arteries involved,[20] which has now been assessed in several populations and confirmed.[21] In individuals with early onset CAD, 9p21 is associated with a 50% increased risk in heterozygotes and a twofold risk in homozygotes,[13] which is equivalent to the twofold increased risk in a current smoker,[38] a 40% increased risk of a 10-mm increase in blood pressure,[39] or the 30% increased risk associated with increase LDL-cholesterol.[40] However, using the technique of risk allele counting, Paynter and colleagues[41] did not find any additional risk prediction when adding 9p21 to conventional risk. Similarly, estimating the number of risk variants per individual, Ripatti and colleagues[42] determined whether such scoring would improve diagnostic ability beyond standard risk algorithms. Although a comparison of those with the upper-most quintile versus the lower-most quintile of genetic risk score conferred a relative risk of 1.7, genetic risk scoring did not improve the C index over traditional risk factors and family history. Moreover, it did not affect net reclassification movement.[42]

Both studies used mere allele counting to generate their scores, thereby potentially blunting the effects of more important SNPs, such as 9p21. Secondly, both studies omitted important SNPs that have been demonstrated to contribute to CAD heritability. Furthermore, discoveries through GWAS to date are not sufficient to account for the estimated heritable component of CAD; the genetics that underlie the missing hereditability of CAD remains to be defined.[43] In contrast, Davies and colleagues,[44] using a weighted genetic risk score and logistic regression, assessed the effect of combining 9p21 with 11 other genetic variants and showed improvement in risk prediction; however, the effect was modest. Talmud and colleagues,[45] in a longitudinal study, showed 9p21 had a modest effect and did reclassify a significant number of individuals into different risk categories. Routine genetic screening is probably not recommended until it has been proved that the results will alter patient management. It is to be realized, however, that the technological barrier of promptly genotyping multiple genetic variants no longer exists. Hundreds of genotypes can be analyzed, with interpretational results, within an hour.

A major impact from genetic variants is likely to be on the development of novel therapy. Emphasis must be on the observation that 22 of the 30 genetic variants act through mechanisms independent of known risk factors. Although cholesterol dominates the prevention and treatment of CAD today, it is unlikely that such dominance will remain in a few years. It would be reasonable to assume that one or more of these mechanisms will take its place along with cholesterol in dominating prevention and treatment in the future.

## SUMMARY

The next decade will focus on identifying the missing heritability of CAD. This process will involve a more comprehensive interrogation of common SNPs that impart modest biologic effect and an interrogation of rare SNPs that impart profound biologic effect. In parallel, a continued investigation of the underlying biology of the described association will likely yield novel pathways that would provide therapeutic targets.

Furthermore, once we obtain a more complete inventory of sequence variation that predisposes to CAD, a more realistic assessment of the role of genetic risk scoring allied with standard risk algorithms will be possible. This assessment would be facilitated by more nuanced phenotyping of CAD cases in GWAS. Also, a continued effort to catalog genetic variation that determines drug response and the propensity for adverse side effects is imperative. In concert, this will facilitate a transition to a more personalized brand of medicine.

## REFERENCES

1. Murray CJ, Lopez AD. Global mortality, disability, and the contribution of risk factors: Global Burden of Disease Study. Lancet 1997;349(9063):1436–42.
2. Venter JC, Adams MD, Myers EW, et al. The sequence of the human genome. Science 2001;291:1304–51.

3. Rodriguez-Campos A, Azorin F. RNA is an integral component of chromatin that contributes to its structural organization. PLos One 2007;2(11):e1182.
4. Small EM, Frost RJA, Olson E. MicroRNAs add a new dimension to Cardiovascular Disease. Circulation 2010;121:1022–32.
5. Stranger BEFM, Dunning M, Ingle CE, et al. Relative impact of nucleotide and copy number variation on gene expression phenotypes. Science 2007; 315(5813):848–53.
6. The International HapMap Consortium. The International HapMap Project. Science 2003;426:789–96.
7. Hirshhorn JN, Daly MJ. Genome-wide Association Studies for Common Diseases and Complex Traits. Nat Rev Genet 2005;6:95–108.
8. Brown MS, Goldstein JL. Familial hypercholesterolemia: A genetic defect in the low-density lipoprotein receptor. N Engl J Med 1976;294(25):1386–90.
9. Hedley PL, Jorgensen P, Schlamowitz S, et al. The genetic basis of long QT and short QT syndromes: a mutation update. Hum Mutat 2009;30(11):1486–511.
10. Wang L, Seidman JG, Seidman CE. Narrative review: harnessing molecular genetics for the diagnosis and management of hypertrophic cardiomyopathy. Ann Intern Med 2010;152(8):513–20, W181.
11. Gollob MH, Green MS, Tang AS, et al. Identification of a gene responsible for familial Wolff-Parkinson-White syndrome. N Engl J Med 2001;344(24):1823–31.
12. McPherson R, Pertsemlidis A, Kavaslar N, et al. A common allele on chromosome 9 associated with coronary heart disease. Science 2007;316(5830):1488–91.
13. Helgadottir A, Thorleifsson G, Manolescu A, et al. A Common Variant on Chromosome 9p21 affects the risk of Myocardial Infarction. Science 2007;316(5830): 1491–3.
14. Samani NJ, Erdmann J, Hall AS, et al. Genome-wide Association Analysis of Coronary Artery Disease. New Engl J Med 2007;357(5):443–53.
15. Ding H, Xu Y, Wang X, et al. 9p21 is a Shared Susceptibility Locus Strongly for Coronary Artery Disease and Weakly for Ischemic Stroke in Chinese Han Population. Circ Cardiovasc Genet 2009;2(4):338–46.
16. Hinohara K, Nakajima T, Takahashi M, et al. Replication of the association between a chromosome 9p21 polymorphism and coronary artery disease in Japanese and Korean populations. J Hum Genet 2008;53(4):357–9.
17. A genome-wide association study in Europeans and South Asians identifies five new loci for coronary artery disease. Nat Genet 2011;43(4):339–44.
18. Assimes TL, Knowles JW, Basu A, et al. Susceptibility locus for clinical and subclinical coronary artery disease at chromosome 9p21 in the multi-ethnic ADVANCE study. Hum Mol Genet 2008;17(15):2320–8.
19. Helgadottir A, Thorleifsson G, Magnusson KP, et al. The same sequence variant on 9p21 associates with myocardial infarction, abdominal aortic aneurysm and intracranial aneurysm. Nat Genet 2008;40(2):217–24.
20. Dandona S, Stewart AF, Chen L, et al. Gene dosage of the common variant 9p21 predicts severity of coronary artery disease. J Am Coll Cardiol 2010;56(6):479–86.
21. Ardissino D, Berzuini C, Merlini PA, et al. Influence of 9p21.3 Genetic Variants on Clinical and Angiographic Outcomes in Early-Onset Myocardial Infarction. JACC 2011;58(4):426–34.
22. Jarinova O, Stewart AF, Roberts R, et al. Functional analysis of the chromosome 9p21.3 coronary artery disease risk locus. Arterioscler Thromb Vasc Biol 2009; 29(10):1671–7.
23. Visel A, Zhu Y, May D, et al. Targeted deletion of the 9p21 non-coding coronary artery disease risk interval in mice. Nature 2010;464(7287):409–12.

24. Harismendy O, Notani D, Song X, et al. 9p21 DNA variants associated with coronary artery disease impair interferon-y signalling response. Nature 2011; 470(7333):264–8.
25. Kathiresan S, Voight BF, Purcell S, et al. Genome-wide association of early-onset myocardial infarction with single nucleotide polymorphisms and copy number variants. Nature Genetics 2009;41(3):334–41.
26. Erdmann J, Groszhennig A, Braund PS, et al. New susceptibility locus for coronary artery disease on chromosome 3q22.3. Nat Genet 2009;41(3):280–2.
27. Tregouet DA, Konig IR, Erdmann J, et al. Genome-wide haplotype association study identifies the SLC22A3-LPAL2-LPA gene cluster as a risk locus for coronary artery disease. Nat Genet 2009;41(3):283–5.
28. Schunkert H, Konig IR, Kathiresan S, et al. Large-scale association analysis identifies 13 new susceptibility loci for coronary artery disease. Nat Genet 2011;43(4): 333–8.
29. Wang F, Xu CQ, He Q, et al. Genome-wide association identifies a susceptibility locus for coronary artery disease in the Chinese Han population. Nat Genet 2011; 43(4):345–9.
30. Preuss M, Konig IR, Thompson JR, et al. Design of the Coronary ARtery DIsease Genome-Wide Replication And Meta-Analysis (CARDIoGRAM) Study: A Genome-wide association meta-analysis involving more than 22 000 cases and 60 000 controls. Circ Cardiovasc Genet 2010;3(5):475–83.
31. Reilly MP, Li M, He J, et al. Identification of ADAMTS7 as a novel locus for coronary atherosclerosis and association of ABO with myocardial infarction in the presence of coronary atherosclerosis: two genome-wide association studies. Lancet 2011;377(9763):383–92.
32. Musunuru K, Strong A, Frank-Kamenetsky M, et al. From noncoding variant to phenotype via SORT1 at the 1p13 cholesterol locus. Nature 2010;466(7307): 714–9.
33. Mega JL, Close SL, Wiviott SD, et al. Cytochrome p-450 polymorphisms and response to clopidogrel. N Engl J Med 2009;360(4):354–62.
34. Mega JL, Close SL, Wiviott SD, et al. Cytochrome P450 genetic polymorphisms and the response to prasugrel: relationship to pharmacokinetic, pharmacodynamic, and clinical outcomes. Circulation 2009;119(19):2553–60.
35. Rieder MJ, Reiner AP, Gage BF, et al. Effect of VKORC1 haplotypes on transcriptional regulation and warfarin dose. N Engl J Med 2005;352(22):2285–93.
36. Epstein RS, Moyer TP, Aubert RE, et al. Warfarin genotyping reduces hospitalization rates results from the MM-WES (Medco-Mayo Warfarin Effectiveness study). J Am Coll Cardiol 2010;55(25):2804–12.
37. Link E, Parish S, Armitage J, et al. SLCO1B1 variants and statin-induced myopathy–a genomewide study. N Engl J Med 2008;359(8):789–99.
38. Schaefer EJ, Lamon-Fava S, Jenner JL, et al. Lipoprotein(a) levels and risk of coronary heart disease in men. The lipid Research Clinics Coronary Primary Prevention Trial. JAMA 1994;271(13):999–1003.
39. Sesso HD, Stampfer MJ, Rosner B, et al. Systolic and Diastolic Blood Pressure, Pulse Pressure, and Mean Arterial Pressure as Predictors of Cardiovascular Disease Risk in Men. Hypertension 2000;36(5):801–7.
40. The Emerging Risk Factors Collaboration. Major Lipids, Apolipoproteins, and Risk of Vascular Disease. JAMA: The Journal of the American Medical Association 2009;302(18):1993–2000.
41. Paynter NP, Chasman DI, Pare G, et al. Association between a literature-based genetic risk score and cardiovascular events in women. JAMA 2010;303:631–7.

42. Ripatti S, Tikkanen E, Orho-Melander M, et al. A multilocus genetic risk score for coronary heart disease: case-control and prospective cohort analyses. The Lancet 2010;376(9750):1393–400.

43. Manolio TA, Collins FS, Cox NJ, et al. Finding the missing heritability of complex diseases. Nature 2009;461:747–53.

44. Davies RW, Dandona S, Stewart AF, et al. Improved prediction of cardiovascular disease based on a panel of single nucleotide polymorphisms identified through genome-wide association studies. Circ Cardiovasc Genet 2010;3(5):468–74.

45. Talmud PJ, Cooper JA, Palmen J, et al. Chromosome 9p21.3 Coronary Heart Disease Locus Genotype and Prospective Risk of CHD in Healthy Middle-Aged Men. Clinical Chemistry 2008;54(3):467–74.

# Statins Personalized

H. Robert Superko, MD[a,b,c],*, Kathryn M. Momary, PharmD, BCPS[b],
Yonghong Li, PhD[a]

**KEYWORDS**

- Genetic • Cholesterol • Statin • Coronary heart disease
- Polymorphism

Statins are among the most widely used medications in the Western world. The percentage of adults 45 years of age and over using statin drugs has increased from 2.4% from 1988 to 1994 to 25.1% from 2005 to 2008.[1] Despite effective low-density-lipoprotein cholesterol (LDL-C) reduction with these compounds, a large amount of residual risk remains in patients treated with statins. For example, in randomized placebo controlled trials a mean 27% relative risk reduction equates to a 3.4% absolute risk reduction.[2]

One possible explanation for the large residual risk following statin therapy may be the heterogeneity of statin responsiveness within the human population. Patients may differ in three ways: (1) the effect of statins on lipoprotein metabolism and, primarily, LDL-C reduction; (2) the response to statin therapy in terms of clinical event benefit, which may be independent of the lipoprotein response; and (3) the adverse effects attributed to statin use.

The cholesterol pathway has become greatly clarified in the 20 years since the elucidation of the regulation of 3-hydroxy-3-methylglutaryl coenzyme A (HMG-CoA) reductase (direct target of statins) by Goldstein and Brown.[3] This pathway involves cholesterol biosynthesis, transcription regulation of cholesterol homeostasis, cholesterol esterification and ester hydrolysis, dietary absorption, bile acid metabolism and steroid hormone production. Five major enzymes play a role in basic lipid metabolism: lipoprotein lipase (LPL), hepatic lipase (HL), endothelial lipase (EL), lecithin-cholesterol acyltransferase (LCAT), and acyl-CoA:cholesterol acyltransferase (ACAT). LPL is

Financial Disclosure and Conflict of Interest: Drs Superko and Li are employees of Celera Corporation. Celera is a gene discovery company and provides genetic testing services through Quest Diagnostics and Berkeley HeartLab. Drs Superko and Li own no stock and have no stock options in Quest Diagnostics, Celera, or Berkeley HeartLab. Dr Momary has an investigator-initiated grant from Pfizer.

[a] Celera Corporation, 1401 Harbor Bay Parkway, Alameda, CA 94502, USA
[b] Mercer University College of Pharmacy and Health Sciences, 3001 Mercer University Drive, Atlanta, GA 30341-4415, USA
[c] Saint Joseph's Hospital of Atlanta, Atlanta, 5665 Peachtree Dunwoody Road, Atlanta, GA 30342, USA
* Corresponding author. Celera Corporation, 1401 Harbor Bay Parkway, Alameda, CA 94502.
E-mail address: Robert.Superko@celera.com

a lipolytic enzyme located on the surface of vascular endothelial cells and macrophages, and apolipoprotein (apo) C-II is a cofactor for LPL action. HL is an enzyme synthesized by hepatocytes that binds to endothelial cells and, in conjunction with cholesteryl ester transfer protein (CETP) activity, is believed to reduce the core of large high-density lipoprotein (HDL) HDL2 particles. EL is a lipolytic enzyme that uses phospholipids as the substrate. LCAT is responsible for the esterification of cholesterol molecules in HDL. ACAT serves to convert free cholesterol to esterified cholesterol intracellularly. CETP mediates the exchange of triglycerides from very-low-density lipoprotein (VLDL) or low-density lipoprotein (LDL) particles for cholesterol ester in HDL particles.

Membrane modulators affect the ability of cholesterol to enter or leave the cell. The ATP-binding cassette transporter 1 is a protein that plays a role in reverse cholesterol transport through transmembrane lipid transport.[4] Apoproteins are proteins attached to a lipid particle that can be recognized by a receptor and assist in uptake or activation of cellular mechanisms.[5] Apo B serves as an identification protein for specific receptors located on hepatic and peripheral cells involved with lipoprotein metabolism. Apo C, along with apo A-I, is an activator of LCAT. The hydrolysis of triglycerides by LPL is dependent on apo C-II. Apo E plays an important role in hepatic clearance of VLDL remnants and HDL recognition, and defects in apo E lead to increased plasma cholesterol and triglycerides and increased risk of developing atherosclerosis.[6]

Blood lipid levels are expected to be modulated by genetic variants that alter the function and activity of the molecules in lipid and cholesterol pathways. These genetic variants and others that affect statin pharmacokinetics may also affect statin responsiveness. This article reviews the recent genetic studies of lipid levels and statin responsiveness, focusing on those with the most compelling biologic and statistical evidence.

## GENETIC CONTRIBUTORS TO BLOOD LIPID LEVELS

Plasma lipid levels are highly heritable traits: more than 50% interindividual variation in LDL-C levels is attributed to genetic factors.[7] Many genetic contributors to plasma lipid levels have been revealed in studies of Mendelian lipid disorders in families and association studies of lipid levels in the general population. Mendelian lipid disorders result from mutations of severe functional consequence in single genes, whereas variation in lipid levels in the general population is thought to be modulated by genetic variants of weak-to-moderate effect in multiple genes. Among the most notable discoveries from Mendelian studies are genetic mutations in the LDL receptor (LDLR) that cause elevated LDL-C levels and early-onset coronary heart disease (CHD).[8] A recent genome-wide association study (GWAS)[9] has identified variants at 95 genetic loci associated with lipid levels. This GWAS tested approximately 2.6 million single-nucleotide polymorphisms (SNPs) across the genome for association with lipid levels in over 100,000 individuals of European ancestry. The 95 lipid-associated loci include some that had been identified from the Mendelian studies[10] and all that had been identified from a spate of previous GWAS that had tested fewer SNPs and studied fewer participants.[11–19] Thirty-seven of the GWAS loci are associated with LDL-C levels (**Fig. 1**), 47 with HDL-C levels, and 32 with triglyceride (TG) levels. Some of the GWAS loci are associated with more than one lipid trait (eg, apo B gene *APOB* with HDL-C and TG, and the apo A-1 gene *APOA1* cluster with LDL-C, HDL-C and TG). Some, particularly those associated with LDL-C levels, are also associated with CHD.[9,11,19,20]

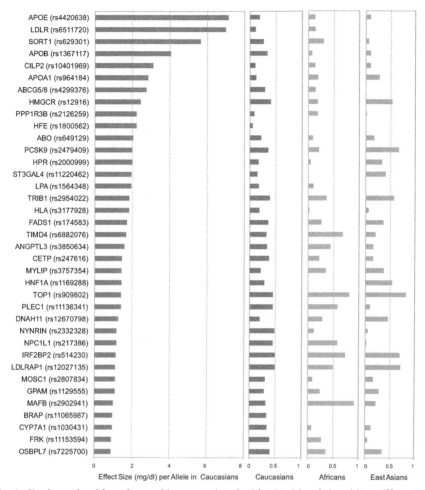

**Fig. 1.** Single nucleotide polymorphisms associated with LDL-C levels in whites. Effect sizes are for each copy of the minor allele, compared with the major allele, and are presented in absolute values for the purpose of between SNP comparisons. Data were extracted from the supplementary Table 1 in Teslovich and colleagues.[9] The three right-most panels show allele frequency in various ethnicities. Data were based on the HapMap results (www.hapmap. org). Note that SNPs associated with LDL-C levels in whites may be not polymorphic in other ethnicities (eg, rs6511720 of LDLR in East Asians) and, even if with similar frequencies, may be not associated with LDL-C levels in other ethnicities (eg, rs4420638 of APOE in African Americans[26]).

The GWAS studies identified many genes that, based on substantial biologic and genetic evidence, were already thought to be involved in lipid metabolism and regulation. For example, the apo E (*APOE*) ε4 variant is in moderate linkage disequilibrium with rs4420638 ($r^2$ = 0.71),[20] which had the largest effect size on LDL-C levels (see **Fig. 1**).[9] Therefore, association of rs4420638 with LDL-C levels is likely due to the association of common apo E isoforms (ε2, ε3, and ε4) with LDL-C levels. The effect of apo E isoforms on LDL-C levels has been demonstrated in many previous studies[21] and in a meta-analysis with approximately 61,000 individuals[22]: carriers of the ε2 genotype have the lowest LDL-C levels and carriers of the ε4 genotype have the highest LDL-C levels (**Fig. 2**). In addition to *APOE*, several other genes are also known to be involved in lipid metabolism; noticeable examples for LDL-C metabolism include *LDLR*, *APOB*, *APOA1*, *HMGCR* (encoding HMG-CoA reductase), and *PCSK9* (encoding proprotein convertase subtilisin/kexin type 9).

The GWAS findings, together with subsequent functional characterization,[9,23] have also revealed several novel genes with roles in regulating lipid levels. For example, an intronic SNP in *GALNT2* (encoding UDP-N-acetyl-α-D-galactosamine:polypeptide N-acetylgalactosaminyl transferase 2) is associated with HDL-C levels. Overexpression of *GALNT2* decreases plasma HDL-C levels in mouse liver whereas knockdown of *GALNT2* increases plasma HDL-C levels, indicating that GALNT2 is directly

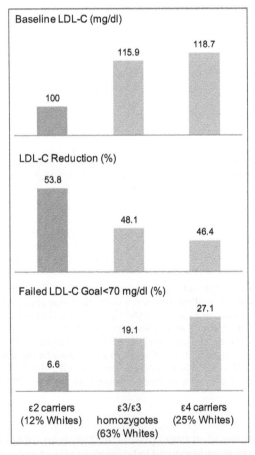

**Fig. 2.** Baseline LDL-C levels and reduction in LDL-C levels and proportion of individuals who did not reach the LDL-C level less than 70 mg/dL among the acute coronary syndrome patients treated with 80 mg/d atorvastatin for 30 days in the PROVE IT-TIMI 22 trial according to APOE genotype. Frequencies of individual APOE genotypes among the white participants in the study are listed in the parenthesis. (*Data from* Mega JL, Morrow DA, Brown A, et al. Identification of genetic variants associated with response to statin therapy. Arterioscler Thromb Vasc Biol 2009;29(9):1310–5.)

involved in HDL-C metabolism.[9] Similarly, *SORT1* (encoding sortilin 1, a multiligand type-1 receptor homologous to the yeast carboxypeptidase Y sorting receptor VPS10 protein) is now known to be a regulator of LDL-C levels for: (1) several SNPs at the locus, including rs12740374, which alters the binding site for CCAAT/enhancer-binding protein (C/EBP) transcription factors, are associated with LDL-C levels; (2) levels of *SORT1* transcripts are affected by the genotype of rs12740374 in humans; and (3) overexpression and knockdown of *SORT1* in mice result in decreased and increased levels of LDL-C, respectively.[23]

Further genetic studies can help to more fully take the advantage of these GWAS findings to better predict, prevent, and treat cardiovascular diseases. One study would be to fine map and resequence the lipid-associated loci. The known genetic variants combined do not fully account for genetic variation in plasma lipid levels in the general population. For example, only a quarter of variation in LDL-C levels could be explained by the known LDL-C–associated SNPs combined.[9] Some of the missing genetic heritability may lie in the lipid-associated genes in GWAS and these unidentified variants may be independent from the initial hits and/or are rare.[24] These genetic variants may be uncovered by fine mapping and resequencing. Rare genetic variants may be associated with larger effects on blood lipid levels than common variants. The common variants identified in GWAS have predictably modest effect on lipid levels. For example, each of the minor alleles of the top four SNPs is associated with a change of LDL-C levels by about 4 to 8 mg/dL in whites. The effect size associated with most other SNPs is less than 2 mg/dL (see **Fig. 1**). These effect sizes are in stark contrast to those of familiar mutations. For example, a missense mutation (V408M) in *LDLR* results in a change of approximately 120 mg/dL in plasma LDL-C level.[25] Another study would be to determine the gene-environment effects of both common and rare variants on lipid levels. Environmental factors such as diet composition may interact with a genotype that results in a variable genotypic expression. These studies should be performed in multiple ethnic groups because of ethnic variability. The alleles associated with blood lipid levels in whites vary in frequency among ethnic groups (see **Fig. 1**). Therefore, their contribution to blood lipid levels will vary among these groups. For example, four SNPs associated with LDL-C levels in whites (including rs6511720 in *LDLR,* which had the second largest effect in whites) have not been found in East Asians, and the minor alleles of many other SNPs (eg, rs217386 in *NPC1L1*) are less frequent in East Asians than in whites. In general, however, most of the SNPs associated with lipid levels in whites are applicable to other ethnic groups.[9,26]

## PHENOTYPE AND STATIN RESPONSE

Although statins can reduce average LDL-C levels by as much as 60%,[27] the magnitude of LDL-C reduction from statin therapy varies from person to person.[28] Phenotypic and demographic characteristics can affect the blood lipid and clinical event response to statin therapy. Compliance to the medication regimen seems to be the most important nongenetic contributor to statin response. An Italian study has reported that, in a primary prevention population, only 19% of patients were adherent to the regimen. For secondary prevention patients, only 41% took the statin more than 80% of the time.[29] Compliance is reflected in blood lipid levels. For example, the mean reduction in LDL-C following treatment with 80 mg/d lovastatin has been reported to be 41.9% with full compliance compared with 20.3% with 80% compliance in the Expanded Clinical Evaluation of Lovastatin (EXCEL) study.[30] Numerous environmental issues have been reported to adversely affect statin compliance. These include younger age, primary versus secondary prevention, number of daily drug doses, female gender, higher co-pay, and a rural living environment.[29,31,32]

Age and ethnicity may also influence LDL-C reduction from statin therapy. In the Cholesterol and Pharmacogenetics (CAP) trial, LDL-C reduction from simvastatin therapy was greater among older subjects compared with young ones.[33] The older patients, compared with the younger ones, also received greater LDL-C reduction from pravastatin therapy in the Long-Term Intervention with Pravastatin in Ischemic Disease (LIPID) study,[34] the Cholesterol and Recurrent Events (CARE) trial,[35] and from lovastatin therapy in the EXCEL study.[30] In a retrospective cohort study, the probability of attaining the LDL-C goal, following the use of statins, increased with age.[36] However, another pooled retrospective analysis found consistent lipid-lowering effect from ezetimibe/simvastatin across age as well as other demographic information including ethnicity.[37] Although no difference in LDL-C reduction from atorvastatin therapy was observed in a South Asian population compared with a white population,[38] there seems to be some small variation in LDL-C reduction from statins between whites and African Americans.[30,33] In response to 40 mg/d simvastatin in a study of 944 subjects, whites had a 3 mg/dL greater reduction in LDL-C compared with African Americans[33] and, in response to 80 mg/d lovastatin, whites revealed a 40.9% reduction in LDL-C level compared with 38.0% in African Americans.[30]

The effect of other phenotypic and demographic characteristics on lipid lowering from statin therapy has also been investigated. Higher LDL-C values before the start of statin therapy were associated with greater LDL-C reduction following statin treatment compared with subjects with lower baseline LDL-C.[39] Nonsmokers were reported to have larger LDL-C reduction in response to statin therapy compared with smokers.[33] Subjects with low plasma triglyceride levels were reported to have larger LDL-C reduction compared with subjects with elevated triglycerides.[40] Low alcohol consumption was associated with greater LDL-C reduction from pravastatin therapy.[40] Postmenopausal women treated with simvastatin achieved significantly greater LDL-C reduction compared with men (-28% vs -20%, respectively) when the dose effect was calibrated by body weight.[41] However, further studies in these areas are needed because these effects were not consistent across a limited number of studies.[33,37,42]

## GENETIC CONTRIBUTORS TO STATIN-INDUCED LDL-C REDUCTION

Response to statin therapy is also affected by genetic factors. Recent GWAS studies of LDL-C reduction from statin therapy suggest that multiple genetic loci with small individual contribution are in play.[43,44] The first GWAS study of atorvastatin-treated subjects from the Treating to New Target (TNT) trial, which tested approximately 300,000 SNPs in nearly 2000 individuals, failed to identify SNPs with genome-wide significance ($P<5 \times 10^{-8}$).[43] A subsequent meta-analysis of three GWAS studies of approximately 3900 subjects from the TNT trial, the CAP trial, and the Pravastatin Inflammation/CRP Evaluation (PRINCE) trial did not yield any SNPs that were significantly associated with differential LDL-C reduction.[44] Notwithstanding incomplete coverage on genetic variation across genome by these GWAS, these results underscore the supposition that variation in LDL-C reduction from statin therapy is genetically complex.

Genetic variants affecting lipid and cholesterol metabolism and statin pharmacokinetics have strong a priori plausibility to modulate LDL-C reduction from statin therapy. Several candidate genes have been investigated before recent GWAS[28] and, although many candidate gene studies are inconclusive, there is now indisputable evidence for the association of LDL-C reduction from statin therapy with

*APOE*. Interesting evidence for the association of LDL-C reduction from statin therapy with *HMGCR* and *SLCO1B1* (encoding OATP1B1 or organic anion transporter polypeptide 1B1) also merits discussion.

Association of LDL-C reduction from statin therapy with common APOE variants has been consistently demonstrated in studies with large numbers of subjects.[21,43,45] These studies, and others,[46–50] generally show that *APOE* ε4 carriers, compared with noncarriers, have less reduction in LDL-C from statin therapy (see **Fig. 2**). For example, rs7412, which is one of the two SNPs that define common *APOE* variants, was associated with LDL-C reduction from statin therapy in the TNT trial ($P = 6 \times 10^{-30}$),[43] in the Statin Response Examined by Genetic Haplotype Markers (STRENGTH) study ($P = .009$),[45] and in the Pravastatin or Atorvastatin Evaluation and Infection Therapy—Thrombolysis In Myocardial Infarction 22 (PROVE IT–TIMI22) study ($P = 8.3 \times 10^{-6}$ for atorvastatin and 0.00065 for pravastatin).[21] In the TNT trial, the relative reduction in LDL-C levels from 80 mg/d atorvastatin was 46.4% among *APOE* ε4 carriers and 53.8% among APOE ε2 carriers.[21] This finding is clinically interesting because *APOE* ε4 carriers, compared with noncarriers, also have higher LDL-C levels at baseline (see **Fig. 2**). The dual effect of *APOE* ε4 genotype on baseline LDL-C levels and LDL-C reduction from statins is most conspicuously illustrated when assessing whether targeted LDL-C levels are reached from statin therapy. For example, among patients treated with 80 mg/d atorvastatin in the PROVE IT–TIMI22 study, more than a quarter of *APOE* ε4 carriers failed to achieve the LDL-C goal of less than 70 mg/d whereas less than a tenth of APOE ε2 carriers failed the same goal[21] (see **Fig. 2**). Among patients treated with 40 mg/d pravastatin in the PROVE IT–TIMI22 study, nearly 80% *APOE* ε4 carriers failed to achieve the LDL-C goal of less than 70 mg/d whereas approximately 55% APOE ε2 carriers failed the same goal.[21] A clinical implication from this finding is that, to reach the LDL-C target of less than 70 mg/dL (optional goal for individuals with high cardiovascular risk), *APOE* ε4 carriers will more likely need to (1) be on intensive statin therapy and (2) use additional LDL-C lowering methods (diet, combinational therapy, etc).

Statins inhibit cholesterol biosynthesis by directly targeting its rate-limiting enzyme HMG-CoA reductase, which is encoded by the *HMGCR* gene. However, reports have been mixed regarding whether polymorphisms in *HMGCR* affect LDL-C reduction from statin therapy.[43,45,49,51–54] Two highly correlated SNPs (rs17244841 and rs17238540; $r^2 = 0.90$) were initially found to associate with LDL-C reduction from statin therapy in the PRINCE study[51]; carriers of the minor allele of these SNPs, compared with noncarriers, had smaller LDL-C reduction from 40 mg/d pravastatin. Association of the minor allele of rs17244841 with attenuated LDL-C reduction from 40 mg/d simvastatin was also observed in the CAP trial and, in this study, a haplotype (H7) consisting of rs17244841, rs384662, and rs17238540 was associated with LDL-C reduction from statin therapy in black (but not white) patients.[52] An SNP tightly linked to rs384662 (rs12916, $r^2 = 1.0$) was also associated with LDL-C reduction from statin therapy in a Chinese cross-sectional study.[55] However, unlike these positive association studies, rs17238540 was not associated with LDL-C reduction from pravastatin in the Prospective Study of Pravastatin in the Elderly at Risk (PROSPER),[53] from pravastatin in the Atorvastatin Comparative Cholesterol Efficacy and Safety Study (ACCESS),[49] or from atorvastatin in the TNT trial,[43] and rs77244841 was not associated with LDL-C reduction from statin therapy in the STRENGTH study.[45] In addition, neither rs17238540 nor rs77244841 was associated with LDL-C reduction from fluvastatin therapy in the Assessment of Lescol in Renal Transplantation (ALERT) Study.[54] These inconsistent findings prevent a firm conclusion regarding a role of the *HMGCR* variants in LDL-C reduction from statin therapy. However, alleles at rs384662 within the H7 haplotype differentially affect alternative splicing of exon 13 of *HMGCR* mRNA.[56,57] Specifically, the minor allele of rs384662 is associated with increased expression of alternatively spliced *HMGCR* transcript lacking exon 13 and, possibly thereby, with lower sensitivity to statin inhibition. Given this attractive biologic rationale and low power of reported studies for low frequent variants such as rs17238540 (which had a minor allele frequency of ~2.0% in the PROSPER population), additional large studies are warranted to determine whether these *HMGCR* variants are associated with LDL-C reduction from statin therapy. Several other SNPs in *HMGCR* were also reported to be associated with LDL-C reduction from statin therapy in the TNT trial[43] and to merit further investigation.

Most statins are transported by OATP1B1 into hepatocytes,[58] where they inhibit the conversion of 3-hydroxy-3-methylglutaryl coenzyme A to mevalonate during cholesterol biosynthesis. Therefore, genetic variants that affect the influx activity of OATP1B1 have the potential to affect the concentration of statins in hepatocytes and consequently the ability of statins to lower LDL-C levels. One such functional variant is rs4149056 in the *SLCO1B1* gene, which encodes either an alanine (commonly referred to as the *5 allele) or the more common valine variant at position 174 of the OATP1B1 polypeptide. The Val174 to Ala substitution alters the trafficking of OATP1B1 polypeptide to the cell surface, resulting in lower transporter activity in carriers of the *5 allele than in noncarriers.[59] As expected, the *5 allele is associated with increased plasma concentration of atorvastatin,[60] rosuvastatin,[60] simvastatin,[61] and pravastatin[62] (but not fluvastatin[62]). In over 16,000 participants in the Heart Protection Study (HPS) who received 40 mg/d simvastatin, carriers of the *5 allele, compared with noncarriers, had significantly smaller LDL-C reduction.[63] However, the *5 allele was not associated with LDL-C reduction from statin therapy in a smaller study with approximately 2700 subjects from ACCESS who received various types of statins.[49] The difference in LDL-C reduction from simvastatin therapy in the HPS was, however, modest between carriers of the *5 allele and noncarriers, which may explain inconsistent association between the *5 allele and LDL-C reduction from statin therapy in studies with smaller numbers of participants.[49,58]

## GENETIC CONTRIBUTORS TO STATIN-ASSOCIATED REDUCTION IN CLINICAL EVENTS

Although LDL-C is the primary target of current therapy for individuals at risk of coronary events, LDL-C reduction does not fully capture the benefits from statin therapy in event prevention. Statins are also reported to possess pleiotropic properties, such as antioxidative stress, anti-inflammation, and plague stabilization that contribute to event reduction.[64] These pleiotropic properties provide another level of genetic regulation that may not be adequately assessed in studies that use LDL-C levels as the endpoint. Some recent studies sought to identify genetic variants associated with event reduction from statin therapy (see, for examples, Refs.[43,65–69]). Among these studies, there has been considerable interest and debate for a common SNP (rs20455) in the *KIF6* gene that encodes a member of the kinesin 9 family. This variation leads to an arginine (Arg)-to-tryptophan (Trp) substitution at position 719 (Trp719Arg) of the KIF6 polypeptide. The SNP was associated with risk of coronary events in a meta-analysis of seven large prospective cohort studies,[70] but not with CHD, in a meta-analysis of 16 case-control association studies,[71] in the HPS,[72] or in the Justification for the Use of Statins in Prevention: An Intervention Trial Evaluating Rosuvastatin (JUPITER).[73]

Carriers of the KIF6 719Arg allele have been associated with coronary event reduction from statin therapy in the retrospective analyses of some,[66,74,75] but not other,[72,73] clinical trials. In the CARE trial, the West of Scotland Coronary Prevention Study

(WOSCOPS), and among patients with prior vascular disease in the PROSPER, pravastatin therapy significantly reduced coronary events in carriers of the 719Arg allele, but not in noncarriers.[66,74] In the PROVE IT–TIMI22 study, intensive statin therapy (80 mg/d atorvastatin) resulted in significantly greater reduction in coronary events over moderate statin therapy (40 mg/d pravastatin) in carriers of the 719Arg allele, but not in noncarriers.[75] However, in the HPS, coronary event reduction from simvastatin therapy was at similar levels among carriers of the 719Arg allele and noncarriers.[72] In the JUPITER, coronary event reduction from rosuvastatin therapy, in low-risk subjects, was also at similar levels among carriers of the 719Arg allele and noncarriers.[73] Explanations for these different observations include the possibilities that association of the *KIF6* carrier status with coronary event reduction might be specific to certain statins, limited to certain patient populations, affected by differences in trial design, or a type I error.[72,73]

## GENETIC CONTRIBUTORS TO STATIN-ASSOCIATED ADVERSE EFFECTS

Adverse side effects attributed to statins are rare in clinical trials in which comorbid conditions and multiple drug use are generally excluded; however, muscle discomfort attributed to statin therapy is more common outside of the research setting. Statin-related skeletal muscle complaints range from mild, but troublesome, to disabling myositis with greater than 10-fold elevation in creatine kinase (CK) and, very rarely, fatal rhabdomyolysis. Under these controlled conditions of clinical trials, muscle aches and pains are reported to range between 1% and 7% and severe myopathy is rare at approximately 0.5%.[76] The incidence in the real world, when patients often have comorbidities and multiple drug therapy, may well be higher with as many as 20% of statin users experiencing myopathy in the clinic.[77] Concerns about myopathy has prompted the US Food and Drug Administration (FDA) to recently issue a recommendation to limit the use of the highest approved dose of simvastatin (80 mg/d).[78] Cerivastatin was withdrawn from market completely because it was associated with unacceptably high risk of rhabdomyolysis.[79] Concerns about side effects may have also contributed to poor compliance to statin therapy among those prescribed with the drug ($\sim$ 50% in 6 months[80]) and, consequently, to lower clinical benefit.

Risk factors for statin side effects include demographic and nongenetic factors such as female sex and older age,[77] but genetic factors also significantly contribute to interindividual variation in statin side effects.[81] Rare mutations that cause metabolic myopathies (eg, McArdle disease) have been found to be enriched by a factor as high as 10 among patients with severe statin-induced myopathy.[82] However, a large fraction of genetic variation in statin side effects now seems to be contributed by a polymorphism in the statin transporter gene *SLCO1B1* rs4149056 (Val174Ala).[63]

The *SLCO1B1*\*5 allele (the 174Ala variant) is associated with increased risk of statin side effects. This association was initially observed in a GWAS study in which allele frequencies of approximately 300,000 SNPs were compared between myopathy cases and matched controls; cases were subjects who developed myopathy although controls did not during high-dose (80 mg/d) simvastatin therapy in the Study of the Effectiveness of Additional Reductions in Cholesterol and Homocysteine (SEARCH).[63] Association of myopathy with rs4149056 and a tightly linked SNP, rs4363657 ($r^2 = 0.97$ between the two SNPs), was highly statistically significant (**Table 1**), and the effect associated with the risk allele was strong. Frequencies of the \*5 allele were 45% and 13% in cases and controls, respectively, which translates to a relative risk of 4.5 for carrying one copy of the \*5 allele compared with not carrying the allele. This variant seems to explain a substantial genetic contribution to simvastatin-induced myopathy

**Table 1**
Association of statin-induced side effects with SLCO1B1*5 allele

| Case Definition | Statin | Dose (mg/d) | Risk Ratio (95% CI)[a] | P-Value[a] | Model[b] | References |
|---|---|---|---|---|---|---|
| Myopathy | S | 80 | 4.5 (2.6–7.7) | $2 \times 10^{-9}$ | C vs T | Link et al,[63] 2008 |
| Myopathy | S | 40 | 2.6 (1.3–5.0) | 0.004 | C vs T | Link et al,[63] 2008 |
| Myopathy | A, P, R, S | n/a | 1.5 (0.58–3.69) | 0.21 | CC or TC vs TT | Brunham et al,[84] 2011 |
| Myalgia | A, F, L, P, R, S | 5–80 | 3.5 (0.95–12.6) | 0.073 | CC or TC vs TT | Linde et al,[85] 2010 |
| Adverse Event | A, P, S | 10–80 | 1.7 (1.04–2.8) | 0.03 | CC or TC vs TT | Voora et al,[83] 2009 |
| Statin Intolerance | A, C, F, P, R, S | ≤10–≥160 | 2.05 (1.02–4.09) | 0.043 | CC vs TC or TT | Donnelly et al,[86] 2011 |
| Rhabdomyolysis | C | 0.2–1.6 | 1.89 (1.40–2.56) | $3.6 \times 10^{-5}$ | C vs T | Marciante et al,[87] 2011 |

*Abbreviations:* A, atorva; C, ceriva; F, Fluva; L, lova; P, prava; R, rosuva; S, simva.
[a] 95% CI and 2-sided P-values were directly cited or recalculated (if not reported) from original studies.
[b] The C allele of rs4149056 corresponds to SLCO1B1 174Ala variant and the T allele corresponds to SLCO1B1 Val174 variant.

because 65% of the myopathy cases carried at least one copy of the *5 allele. A replication study in the HPS that compared 40 mg/d simvastatin versus placebo confirmed the association of the *5 allele with increased risk of myopathy: the relative risk of myopathy was 2.6 for simvastatin users carrying one copy of the *5 allele (see **Table 1**).[63]

Subsequent studies further confirmed the association of the SLCO1B1*5 allele with simvastatin-induced myopathy and extended the association to other statins and more common milder statin intolerance (see **Table 1**). The results included the following:

1. In the STRENGTH study, in which participants received atorvastatin, simvastatin, or pravastatin, carriers of the *5 allele, compared with noncarriers, had higher risk of adverse events defined as any side effect, drug discontinuation, myalgia or muscle cramp, or elevated CK levels (adverse effects were predominantly CK-negative).[83] In addition, risk was most pronounced among simvastatin users, moderate among atorvastatin users, and not observed among pravastatin users.
2. In a clinical study, carriers of the *5 allele were also at greater risk of extreme myopathy with CK elevation at greater than 10 times upper limit of the normal.[84] In this study, the risk was observed among simvastatin, but not atorvastatin, users.
3. In another clinical study, carriers of the *5 allele had a threefold increased risk of myalgias ($P = .07$).[85]
4. In patients with a comorbid condition such as type 2 diabetes, homozygous carriers of the *5 allele were at twofold increased risk of general statin intolerance (defined by elevated CK or alanine aminotransferase accompanied by changes in prescription).[86]
5. The *5 allele was also highly significantly associated with rhabdomyolysis in a study of the now-discontinued cerivastatin.[87]

Together, these studies suggest that the *5 allele is associated with broadly defined and commonly observed clinically relevant adverse events caused by multiple statins at different doses.

The consistent association of the SLCO1B1*5 allele with statin-induced myopathy is congruent with the findings that (1) SLCO1B1 is involved in the hepatic transport of statins,[58] (2) the SLCO1B1 174Ala variant has lower transporter activity compared with the Val174 variant,[59] and (3) carriers of the *5 allele have higher plasma concentrations of various statins than noncarriers.[60–62] In fact, before the GWAS study, a rare missense SNP in this gene (rs72661137, corresponding to Trp543Leu) had been suspected to cause pravastatin-induced myopathy in a Japanese patient.[88] In addition to rs4149056 (Val174Ala), another common functional SNP, rs2306283 (Asp130Asn), in SLCO1B1 was also associated with statin intolerance ($P = .03$).[86] However, this SNP was not associated with the risk of rhabdomyolysis[87] and, so far, no other myopathy studies have reported association results for this SNP. Additional studies are needed to ascertain whether this specific genetic variant is also associated with statin-induced myopathy.

The SLCO1B1 genotype information may be used to guide the selection and dosing of statins. Niemi[89] has recently proposed a dosing scheme for various statins according to SLCO1B1 genotype. In general, the maximum doses allowed by the FDA for all individuals (eg, 80 mg/d for simvastatin, atorvastatin, and pravastatin) should be lowered for individuals carrying one copy of the SLCO1B1*5 allele (eg, 40 mg/d for simvastatin, atorvastatin, and pravastatin) and lowered further for individuals carrying two copies of the *5 allele (eg, 20 mg/d for simvastatin and atorvastatin). Because plasma concentrations of fluvastatin did not seem to be affected by the *5 allele,[62] individuals who experience myopathy and are positive for the *5 allele may consider switching to fluvastatin.[89,90] *SLCO1B1* genotype information may help patients who experience myopathy, myalgia, or nonspecific statin associated symptoms to adjust their statin regime. It can also be prognostic of potential side effects, particularly for patients considering high-dose stain therapy.

## SUMMARY

Despite the successful reduction of LDL-C attributed to statin therapy, a large amount of individual variation concerning LDL-C reduction, clinical event reduction, and side effects is evident from clinical trials. Some of this variability is due to nongenetic issues, the most important of which is compliance. However, recent investigations have highlighted clinically relevant polymorphisms that identify subgroups that are more likely to have higher or lower LDL-C at baseline, and a greater or lesser LDL-C response to statin therapy. Some of these polymorphisms are linked to known lipoprotein pathways such as the *APOE* polymorphisms, and some are novel SNPs. However, only about 25% of the variation in LDL-C levels is explained by currently known SNPs underscoring the fact that the genetic effect on statin response is complex. A polymorphism in *SLCO1B1* affects the blood level of some statins and has been linked to statin-associated myopathy, primarily with simvastatin, but also other statins. These genetic polymorphisms that affect statin LDL-C, clinical event response, and side effects seem to be clinically relevant. On-going and future research will allow the individualization of statin therapy, in large part based on genetic polymorphisms.

## ACKNOWLEDGMENTS

We thank Drs James J. Devlin and John J. Sninsky for helpful discussions and comments on this article.

## REFERENCES

1. National Center for Health Statistics. Health, United States, 2010: with special feature on death and dying. Hyattsville (MD); 2011.
2. Superko HR, King S, 3rd. Lipid management to reduce cardiovascular risk: a new strategy is required. Circulation 2008;117(4):560–8 [discussion: 8].
3. Goldstein JL, Brown MS. Regulation of the mevalonate pathway. Nature 1990; 343(6257):425–30.
4. Hamon Y, Broccardo C, Chambenoit O, et al. ABC1 promotes engulfment of apoptotic cells and transbilayer redistribution of phosphatidylserine. Nat Cell Biol 2000;2(7):399–406.
5. Mahley RW, Innerarity TL, Rall SC Jr, et al. Plasma lipoproteins: apolipoprotein structure and function. J Lipid Res 1984;25(12):1277–94.
6. Mahley RW, Innerarity TL, Rall SC Jr, et al. Lipoproteins of special significance in atherosclerosis. Insights provided by studies of type III hyperlipoproteinemia. Ann N Y Acad Sci 1985;454:209–21.
7. Heller DA, de Faire U, Pedersen NL, et al. Genetic and environmental influences on serum lipid levels in twins. N Engl J Med 1993;328(16):1150–6.
8. Hobbs HH, Brown MS, Goldstein JL. Molecular genetics of the LDL receptor gene in familial hypercholesterolemia. Hum Mutat 1992;1(6):445–66.
9. Teslovich TM, Musunuru K, Smith AV, et al. Biological, clinical and population relevance of 95 loci for blood lipids. Nature 2010;466(7307):707–13.
10. Hegele RA. Plasma lipoproteins: genetic influences and clinical implications. Nat Rev Genet 2009;10(2):109–21.

11. Aulchenko YS, Ripatti S, Lindqvist I, et al. Loci influencing lipid levels and coronary heart disease risk in 16 European population cohorts. Nat Genet 2009;41(1): 47–55.

12. Chasman DI, Pare G, Mora S, et al. Forty-three loci associated with plasma lipoprotein size, concentration, and cholesterol content in genome-wide analysis. PLoS Genet 2009;5(11):e1000730.

13. Kathiresan S, Melander O, Guiducci C, et al. Six new loci associated with blood low-density lipoprotein cholesterol, high-density lipoprotein cholesterol or triglycerides in humans. Nat Genet 2008;40(2):189–97.

14. Kathiresan S, Willer CJ, Peloso GM, et al. Common variants at 30 loci contribute to polygenic dyslipidemia. Nat Genet 2009;41(1):56–65.

15. Kooner JS, Chambers JC, Aguilar-Salinas CA, et al. Genome-wide scan identifies variation in MLXIPL associated with plasma triglycerides. Nat Genet 2008;40(2): 149–51.

16. Sabatti C, Service SK, Hartikainen AL, et al. Genome-wide association analysis of metabolic traits in a birth cohort from a founder population. Nat Genet 2009;41(1): 35–46.

17. Sandhu MS, Waterworth DM, Debenham SL, et al. LDL-cholesterol concentrations: a genome-wide association study. Lancet 2008;371(9611):483–91.

18. Wallace C, Newhouse SJ, Braund P, et al. Genome-wide association study identifies genes for biomarkers of cardiovascular disease: serum urate and dyslipidemia. Am J Hum Genet 2008;82(1):139–49.

19. Willer CJ, Sanna S, Jackson AU, et al. Newly identified loci that influence lipid concentrations and risk of coronary artery disease. Nat Genet 2008;40(2):161–9.

20. Waterworth DM, Ricketts SL, Song K, et al. Genetic variants influencing circulating lipid levels and risk of coronary artery disease. Arterioscler Thromb Vasc Biol 2010;30(11):2264–76.

21. Mega JL, Morrow DA, Brown A, et al. Identification of genetic variants associated with response to statin therapy. Arterioscler Thromb Vasc Biol 2009; 29(9):1310–5.

22. Bennet AM, Di Angelantonio E, Ye Z, et al. Association of apolipoprotein E genotypes with lipid levels and coronary risk. JAMA 2007;298(11):1300–11.

23. Musunuru K, Strong A, Frank-Kamenetsky M, et al. From noncoding variant to phenotype via SORT1 at the 1p13 cholesterol locus. Nature 2010;466(7307): 714–9.

24. Manolio TA, Collins FS, Cox NJ, et al. Finding the missing heritability of complex diseases. Nature 2009;461(7265):747–53.

25. Umans-Eckenhausen MA, Sijbrands EJ, Kastelein JJ, et al. Low-density lipoprotein receptor gene mutations and cardiovascular risk in a large genetic cascade screening population. Circulation 2002;106(24):3031–6.

26. Dumitrescu L, Carty CL, Taylor K, et al. Genetic determinants of lipid traits in diverse populations from the population architecture using genomics and epidemiology (PAGE) study. PLoS Genet 2011;7(6):e1002138.

27. Smith ME, Lee NJ, Haney E, et al. Drug class review: HMG-CoA reductase inhibitors (statins) and fixed-dose combination products containing a statin: final report update 5. Portland (OR): Oregon Health & Science University; 2009.

28. Sirtori CR, Mombelli G, Triolo M, et al. Clinical response to statins: Mechanism(s) of variable activity and adverse effects. Ann Med 2011. [Epub ahead of print].

29. Deambrosis P, Saramin C, Terrazzani G, et al. Evaluation of the prescription and utilization patterns of statins in an Italian local health unit during the period 1994–2003. Eur J Clin Pharmacol 2007;63(2):197–203.

30. Shear CL, Franklin FA, Stinnett S, et al. Expanded Clinical Evaluation of Lovastatin (EXCEL) study results. Effect of patient characteristics on lovastatin-induced changes in plasma concentrations of lipids and lipoproteins. Circulation 1992; 85(4):1293–303.
31. Pedan A, Varasteh L, Schneeweiss S. Analysis of factors associated with statin adherence in a hierarchical model considering physician, pharmacy, patient, and prescription characteristics. J Manag Care Pharm 2007;13(6): 487–96.
32. Perreault S, Blais L, Lamarre D, et al. Persistence and determinants of statin therapy among middle-aged patients for primary and secondary prevention. Br J Clin Pharmacol 2005;59(5):564–73.
33. Simon JA, Lin F, Hulley SB, et al. Phenotypic predictors of response to simvastatin therapy among African-Americans and Caucasians: the Cholesterol and Pharmacogenetics (CAP) Study. Am J Cardiol 2006;97(6):843–50.
34. Hunt D, Young P, Simes J, et al. Benefits of pravastatin on cardiovascular events and mortality in older patients with coronary heart disease are equal to or exceed those seen in younger patients: Results from the LIPID trial. Ann Intern Med 2001; 134(10):931–40.
35. Lewis SJ, Moye LA, Sacks FM, et al. Effect of pravastatin on cardiovascular events in older patients with myocardial infarction and cholesterol levels in the average range. Results of the Cholesterol and Recurrent Events (CARE) trial. Ann Intern Med 1998;129(9):681–9.
36. Cone C, Murata G, Myers O. Demographic determinants of response to statin medications. Am J Health Syst Pharm 2011;68(6):511–7.
37. Ose L, Shah A, Davies MJ, et al. Consistency of lipid-altering effects of ezetimibe/ simvastatin across gender, race, age, baseline low density lipoprotein cholesterol levels, and coronary heart disease status: results of a pooled retrospective analysis. Curr Med Res Opin 2006;22(5):823–35.
38. Gupta M, Braga MF, Teoh H, et al. Statin effects on LDL and HDL cholesterol in South Asian and white populations. J Clin Pharmacol 2009;49(7):831–7.
39. de Sauvage Nolting PR, Buirma RJ, Hutten BA, et al. Baseline lipid values partly determine the response to high-dose simvastatin in patients with familial hypercholesterolemia. The examination of probands and relatives in Statin studies with familial hypercholesterolemia (ExPRESS FH). Atherosclerosis 2002;164(2): 347–54.
40. Streja L, Packard CJ, Shepherd J, et al. Factors affecting low-density lipoprotein and high-density lipoprotein cholesterol response to pravastatin in the West Of Scotland Coronary Prevention Study (WOSCOPS). Am J Cardiol 2002;90(7): 731–6.
41. Nakajima K. Sex-related differences in response of plasma lipids to simvastatin: the Saitama Postmenopausal Lipid Intervention Study. S-POLIS Group. Clin Ther 1999;21(12):2047–57.
42. Kannel WB, D'Agostino RB, Stepanians M, et al. Efficacy and tolerability of lovastatin in a six-month study: analysis by gender, age and hypertensive status. Am J Cardiol 1990;66(8):1B–10B.
43. Thompson JF, Hyde CL, Wood LS, et al. Comprehensive whole-genome and candidate gene analysis for response to statin therapy in the treating to new targets (TNT) cohort. Circ Cardiovasc Genet 2009;2:173–81.
44. Barber MJ, Mangravite LM, Hyde CL, et al. Genome-wide association of lipid-lowering response to statins in combined study populations. PLoS One 2010; 5(3):e9763.

45. Voora D, Shah SH, Reed CR, et al. Pharmacogenetic predictors of statin-mediated low-density lipoprotein cholesterol reduction and dose response. Circ Cardiovasc Genet 2008;1:100–6.
46. Ballantyne CM, Herd JA, Stein EA, et al. Apolipoprotein E genotypes and response of plasma lipids and progression-regression of coronary atherosclerosis to lipid-lowering drug therapy. J Am Coll Cardiol 2000;36(5):1572–8.
47. Baptista R, Rebelo M, Decq-Mota J, et al. Apolipoprotein E epsilon-4 polymorphism is associated with younger age at referral to a lipidology clinic and a poorer response to lipid-lowering therapy. Lipids Health Dis 2011;10:48.
48. Donnelly LA, Palmer CN, Whitley AL, et al. Apolipoprotein E genotypes are associated with lipid-lowering responses to statin treatment in diabetes: a Go-DARTS study. Pharmacogenet Genomics 2008;18(4):279–87.
49. Thompson JF, Man M, Johnson KJ, et al. An association study of 43 SNPs in 16 candidate genes with atorvastatin response. Pharmacogenomics J 2005;5(6):352–8.
50. Zintzaras E, Kitsios GD, Triposkiadis F, et al. APOE gene polymorphisms and response to statin therapy. Pharmacogenomics J 2009;9(4):248–57.
51. Chasman DI, Posada D, Subrahmanyan L, et al. Pharmacogenetic study of statin therapy and cholesterol reduction. JAMA 2004;291(23):2821–7.
52. Krauss RM, Mangravite LM, Smith JD, et al. Variation in the 3-hydroxyl-3-methylglutaryl coenzyme a reductase gene is associated with racial differences in low-density lipoprotein cholesterol response to simvastatin treatment. Circulation 2008;117(12):1537–44.
53. Polisecki E, Muallem H, Maeda N, et al. Genetic variation at the LDL receptor and HMG-CoA reductase gene loci, lipid levels, statin response, and cardiovascular disease incidence in PROSPER. Atherosclerosis 2008;200(1):109–14.
54. Singer JB, Holdaas H, Jardine AG, et al. Genetic analysis of fluvastatin response and dyslipidemia in renal transplant recipients. J Lipid Res 2007;48(9):2072–8.
55. Chien KL, Wang KC, Chen YC, et al. Common sequence variants in pharmacodynamic and pharmacokinetic pathway-related genes conferring LDL cholesterol response to statins. Pharmacogenomics 2010;11(3):309–17.
56. Burkhardt R, Kenny EE, Lowe JK, et al. Common SNPs in HMGCR in micronesians and whites associated with LDL-cholesterol levels affect alternative splicing of exon13. Arterioscler Thromb Vasc Biol 2008;28(11):2078–84.
57. Medina MW, Gao F, Ruan W, et al. Alternative splicing of 3-hydroxy-3-methylglutaryl coenzyme A reductase is associated with plasma low-density lipoprotein cholesterol response to simvastatin. Circulation 2008;118(4):355–62.
58. Romaine SP, Bailey KM, Hall AS, et al. The influence of SLCO1B1 (OATP1B1) gene polymorphisms on response to statin therapy. Pharmacogenomics J 2010;10(1):1–11.
59. Tirona RG, Leake BF, Merino G, et al. Polymorphisms in OATP-C: identification of multiple allelic variants associated with altered transport activity among European- and African-Americans. J Biol Chem 2001;276(38):35669–75.
60. Pasanen MK, Fredrikson H, Neuvonen PJ, et al. Different effects of SLCO1B1 polymorphism on the pharmacokinetics of atorvastatin and rosuvastatin. Clin Pharmacol Ther 2007;82(6):726–33.
61. Pasanen MK, Neuvonen M, Neuvonen PJ, et al. SLCO1B1 polymorphism markedly affects the pharmacokinetics of simvastatin acid. Pharmacogenet Genomics 2006;16(12):873–9.
62. Niemi M, Pasanen MK, Neuvonen PJ. SLCO1B1 polymorphism and sex affect the pharmacokinetics of pravastatin but not fluvastatin. Clin Pharmacol Ther 2006; 80(4):356–66.

63. Link E, Parish S, Armitage J, et al. SLCO1B1 variants and statin-induced myopathy—a genomewide study. N Engl J Med 2008;359(8):789–99.
64. Wang CY, Liu PY, Liao JK. Pleiotropic effects of statin therapy: molecular mechanisms and clinical results. Trends Mol Med 2008;14(1):37–44.
65. Hindorff LA, Lemaitre RN, Smith NL, et al. Common genetic variation in six lipid-related and statin-related genes, statin use and risk of incident nonfatal myocardial infarction and stroke. Pharmacogenet Genomics 2008;18(8):677–82.
66. Iakoubova OA, Tong CH, Rowland CM, et al. Association of the Trp719Arg polymorphism in kinesin-like protein 6 with myocardial infarction and coronary heart disease in 2 prospective trials: the CARE and WOSCOPS trials. J Am Coll Cardiol 2008;51(4):435–43.
67. Maitland-van der Zee AH, Peters BJ, Lynch AI, et al. The effect of nine common polymorphisms in coagulation factor genes (F2, F5, F7, F12 and F13) on the effectiveness of statins: the GenHAT study. Pharmacogenet Genomics 2009; 19(5):338–44.
68. Peters BJ, Rodin AS, Klungel OH, et al. Variants of ADAMTS1 modify the effectiveness of statins in reducing the risk of myocardial infarction. Pharmacogenet Genomics 2010;20(12):766–74.
69. Sabatine MS, Ploughman L, Simonsen KL, et al. Association between ADAMTS1 matrix metalloproteinase gene variation, coronary heart disease, and benefit of statin therapy. Arterioscler Thromb Vasc Biol 2008;28(3):562–7.
70. Li Y, Iakoubova O, Shiffman D, et al. KIF6 polymorphism as a predictor of risk of coronary events and of clinical event reduction by statin therapy. Am J Cardiol 2010;106(7):994–8.
71. Assimes TL, Holm H, Kathiresan S, et al. Lack of association between the Trp719Arg polymorphism in kinesin-like protein-6 and coronary artery disease in 19 case-control studies. J Am Coll Cardiol 2010;56(19):1552–63.
72. Hopewell JC, Parish S, Clarke R, et al. No impact of KIF6 genotype on vascular risk and statin response among 18,348 randomized patients in the heart protection study. J Am Coll Cardiol 2011;57(20):2000–7.
73. Ridker PM, Macfadyen JG, Glynn RJ, et al. Kinesin-like protein 6 (KIF6) polymorphism and the Efficacy of rosuvastatin in primary prevention. Circ Cardiovasc Genet 2011;4(3):312–7.
74. Iakoubova OA, Robertson M, Tong CH, et al. KIF6 Trp719Arg polymorphism and effect of statin therapy in elderly patients: results from the PROSPER study. Eur J Cardiovasc Prev Rehabil 2010;17(4):455–61.
75. Iakoubova OA, Sabatine MS, Rowland CM, et al. Polymorphism in KIF6 gene and benefit from statins after acute coronary syndromes: results from the PROVE IT-TIMI 22 study. J Am Coll Cardiol 2008;51(4):449–55.
76. Bays H. Statin safety: an overview and assessment of the data–2005. Am J Cardiol 2006;97(8A):6C–26C.
77. Fernandez G, Spatz ES, Jablecki C, et al. Statin myopathy: a common dilemma not reflected in clinical trials. Cleve Clin J Med 2011;78(6):393–403.
78. Available at: http://www.fda.gov/Drugs/DrugSafety/ucm256581.htm. Accessed September 20, 2011.
79. Available at: http://www.fda.gov/Safety/MedWatch/SafetyInformation/SafetyAlerts forHumanMedicalProducts/ucm172268.htm. Accessed September 20, 2011.
80. National Cholesterol Education Program (NCEP) Expert Panel on Detection E, and Treatment of High Blood Cholesterol in Adults (Adult Treatment Panel III). Third Report of the National Cholesterol Education Program (NCEP) Expert Panel

on Detection, Evaluation, and Treatment of High Blood Cholesterol in Adults (Adult Treatment Panel III) final report. Circulation 2002;106(25):3143–421.

81. Ghatak A, Faheem O, Thompson PD. The genetics of statin-induced myopathy. Atherosclerosis 2010;210(2):337–43.

82. Vladutiu GD, Simmons Z, Isackson PJ, et al. Genetic risk factors associated with lipid-lowering drug-induced myopathies. Muscle Nerve 2006;34(2):153–62.

83. Voora D, Shah SH, Spasojevic I, et al. The SLCO1B1*5 genetic variant is associated with statin-induced side effects. J Am Coll Cardiol 2009;54(17):1609–16.

84. Brunham LR, Lansberg PJ, Zhang L, et al. Differential effect of the rs4149056 variant in SLCO1B1 on myopathy associated with simvastatin and atorvastatin. Pharmacogenomics J 2011. [Epub ahead of print].

85. Linde R, Peng L, Desai M, et al. The role of vitamin D and SLCO1B1*5 gene polymorphism in statin-associated myalgias. Dermatoendocrinol 2010;2(2):77–84.

86. Donnelly LA, Doney AS, Tavendale R, et al. Common nonsynonymous substitutions in SLCO1B1 predispose to statin intolerance in routinely treated individuals with type 2 diabetes: a go-DARTS study. Clin Pharmacol Ther 2011;89(2):210–6.

87. Marciante KD, Durda JP, Heckbert SR, et al. Cerivastatin, genetic variants, and the risk of rhabdomyolysis. Pharmacogenet Genomics 2011;21(5):280–8.

88. Morimoto K, Oishi T, Ueda S, et al. A novel variant allele of OATP-C (SLCO1B1) found in a Japanese patient with pravastatin-induced myopathy. Drug Metab Pharmacokinet 2004;19(6):453–5.

89. Niemi M. Transporter pharmacogenetics and statin toxicity. Clin Pharmacol Ther 2010;87(1):130–3.

90. Peters BJ, Klungel OH, Visseren FL, et al. Pharmacogenomic insights into treatment and management of statin-induced myopathy. Genome Med 2009;1(12):120.

# Childhood Cholesterol Disorders: The Iceberg Base or Nondisease?

Sarah D. de Ferranti, MD, MPH

**KEYWORDS**

- Cholesterol • Prevention • Cardiovascular disease • Screening
- Child • Lipid • Familial hypercholesterolemia

## PEDIATRIC LIPID ABNORMALITIES: SCOPE OF THE PROBLEM

The prevalence of abnormal lipid values in US children and adolescents is high. Analysis of National Health and Nutrition Examination Survey (NHANES) datasets from 1999 to 2006 shows that 20.3% of adolescents aged 12 to 19 years are affected with at least 1 lipid abnormality.[1] Low-density lipoprotein cholesterol (LDL-C) greater than or equal to 130 mg/dL was found in 7.6%, high-density lipoprotein cholesterol (HDL-C) less than or equal to 35 mg/dL in 7.6%; 10.2% of youth aged 12 to 19 years had triglycerides (TG) greater than or equal to 150 mg/dL.[1] There are small gender and racial/ethnic differences in lipid values. Some studies show that girls have slightly higher total cholesterol (TC) and LDL-C than boys, with higher non–HDL-C; newer data suggest that boys are more likely to have lipid abnormalities.[1] Compared with Whites and Asians, African Americans have higher TC and LDL-C but also higher HDL-C; non-HDL-C levels are equivalent.[2,3]

## SIGNIFICANCE OF ATHEROSCLEROSIS DURING CHILDHOOD

Atherosclerosis is the primary cause of cardiovascular disease (CVD); CVD is the most common cause of mortality in adults.[4] The incidence in adults of atherosclerotic events is well described: 406,351 adults died of coronary heart disease in the United States in 2007.[4] Cardiovascular events during adolescence and childhood are not atherosclerotic, except in rare circumstances described below, and are generally related to congenital heart disease or arrhythmias.

The current concept of atherosclerosis is that multiple processes contribute to the vascular disorder. These processes include hyperlipidemia, inflammation, oxidative stress, vessel wall abnormalities, hyperinsulinemia and hyperglycemia, procoaguable states, as well as other less well-defined genetic and environmental elements that are

Department of Cardiology, Children's Hospital Boston, 300 Longwood Avenue, FA607, Boston, MA 02115, USA
*E-mail address:* Sarah.deferranti@cardio.chboston.org

Med Clin N Am 96 (2012) 141–154
doi:10.1016/j.mcna.2012.01.011
0025-7125/12/$ – see front matter © 2012 Elsevier Inc. All rights reserved.

medical.theclinics.com

partially represented by family history. Although autopsy studies of individuals deceased from noncardiovascular causes show that atherosclerosis begins microscopically at the level of the vessel wall,[5,6] it only becomes clinically manifest as insufficient vascular supply to the myocardium, brain, kidney, and skeletal muscle. The pathophysiologic process requires years to reach clinical fruition, and the latency between exposure to risk factors for atherosclerosis and clinical events is decades long in most cases. During childhood, clinical atherosclerotic events are confined to children with rare genetic mutations such as homozygous LDL-C receptor defects (familial hyperlipidemia) or, rarely, those with concomitant medical diseases that accelerate atherosclerosis.

## CHILDHOOD CHOLESTEROL LEVELS AND ATHEROSCLEROSIS

Despite the lack of clinical atherosclerotic events in pediatric populations, the concept that cholesterol is related to atherosclerosis during childhood is supported by several lines of evidence. Most convincing are studies relating the presence of risk factors during childhood to rates of clinical events during adulthood. A few such studies exist. Franks and colleagues[7] examined the Pima Indian population, a group at extremely high risk for diabetes and CVD. Childhood glucose intolerance, obesity, and hypertension were related to death from endogenous causes such as fatty liver, diabetes, and CVD.[7] However, lipid levels were not related to endogenous death in this cohort. This lack of significance could be caused by the normal range of lipids in this population, and the larger effects on mortality of diabetes. The Princeton Lipid Research Clinics follow-up study showed that childhood cardiovascular risk factors predicted non–type 2 diabetes and CVD events 26 years later (6-fold and 14-fold increase in incidence rates).[8]

Other supportive evidence includes the demonstration of a relationship between childhood risk factors and atherosclerosis by pathology. Findings from the Bogalusa (LA) cohort showed associations between childhood CVD risk factors and the extent of atherosclerosis in individuals who died later of accidental causes.[9] In this study, non–HDL-C, LDL-C, TC, and HDL-C all correlated with the presence and degree of vascular involvement. The greater the number of CVD risk factors, as seen in the metabolic syndrome, the more extensive the atherosclerosis on autopsy.[9,10] Similarly, the Pathobiological Determinants of Atherosclerosis in Youth (PDAY) study found lesions in the right coronary artery of ∼25% previously healthy boys and men 15 to 19 years old who died of traumatic causes; the extent of the lesions correlated most strongly with non–HDL-C levels.[6]

Outside of clinical events and pathology studies, studies using preclinical disease by noninvasive testing as the study outcome may be informative. The Muscatine and Bogalusa cohorts show a relationship between childhood risk factors and adult preclinical vascular disease. The Muscatine Study reported that the greater number of metabolic risk factors, the worse the carotid intimal-medial thickness (IMT) and coronary calcium during adulthood.[11,12] A similar relationship was found in the Bogalusa study participants; the presence of more metabolic risk factors during childhood predicted greater femoral IMT in adulthood.[13]

Few intervention trials have been done that would test the relationship between childhood cholesterol and adult CVD. One trial on cholesterol treatment during childhood has been shown to alter preclinical vascular findings.[14] Data from a randomized placebo-controlled trial of pravastatin in children with familial hypercholesterolemia (FH) by Wiegman and colleagues[14] suggested that 2 years of pharmacotherapy to reduce LDL-C could prevent the progression of a combined carotid IMT score. In children who continued on pravastatin for 4.5 more years, IMT continued to differ in the 2 groups despite conversion to treatment in the placebo group, leading the investigators to assert that carotid IMT increases by 0.003 mm in patients with FH for each year that statin therapy is postponed.[15] Earlier initiation of statins was related to less progression of IMT score.[15]

Alterations in lipid values caused by genetic point mutations offer further insight into the relationship between childhood lipid values and CVD. As discussed later, individuals with a clinical picture or genetic diagnosis of FH have higher risks of early atherosclerotic events.[16] These events are related to lifelong exposure to high LDL-C. Conversely, individuals with genetic variants associated with lower LDL-C levels have lower rates of CVD during adulthood. PCSK-9 is a gene encoding the LDL-C receptor. Some genetic variants associated with lack of function of this gene have 15% lower LDL-C levels.[17] Rates of CVD events in individuals with this lack-of-function mutation are decreased by 45%, which is lower than expected given the 15% lower LDL-C level.[17] These findings suggest that lifelong exposure to lower risk factor levels has cumulative effects that may not be achieved by a similar degree of LDL-C lowering that begins in middle age.

## TRACKING OF LIPID DISORDERS FROM CHILDHOOD TO ADULTHOOD

In addition to the evidence described earlier supporting a relationship between childhood cholesterol and atherosclerosis, it is important to know the extent to which childhood cholesterol levels predict adult cholesterol levels. Several studies have examined tracking of lipid values from childhood into adulthood. There are several published studies addressing the issue of tracking that show moderate correlation between childhood and adulthood lipid values.[18–20] The Bogalusa Study (n ≈ 4000) followed children for 12 years.[21] Children with a TC greater than the 75th percentile had a 50% chance of being in the same percentile as adults (twice that expected because of chance). Correlation between childhood and adult TC levels is moderately good (0.44 Beaver County Lipid Study, Young Finns 0.48 to 0.59 for TC, HDL-C, LDL-C).[19,20] In general, higher values and postpubertal testing more strongly predict future lipid values. Extremely increased lipids reliably identify children who are likely to have FH; a TC of greater than 200 mg/dL is 90% specific for FH.[22] Although the correlations are moderate, they do support the concept that modifying the risk factors early may be important and the tracking of cholesterol during development, along with the CVD events, autopsy, preclinical disease, and intervention trial evidence presented earlier, are presented as arguments for childhood lipid screening recommendations.

## SCREENING FOR LIPID DISORDERS

Screening for lipid disorders during childhood has been recommended for more than 2 decades as a means of identifying children at increased risk for early atherosclerosis. In 1986, the American Academy of Pediatrics (AAP) issued the first statement on children and cholesterol.[23] As new literature emerged, there have been regular updates from the National Cholesterol Education Program (NCEP),[24] and the AAP,[25–27] on screening for and treatment of pediatric lipid disorders. The 2008 AAP Cholesterol Statement recommended selective screening based on family history of early atherosclerosis and hyperlipidemia, as well as personal risk factors such as obesity, diabetes, hypertension, and high-risk medical conditions.[27]

The most current guidelines on pediatric cholesterol screening are based on a graded evidence review by the National Heart, Lung, and Blood Institute (NHLBI) Expert Panel on Integrated Guidelines for Cardiovascular Health and Risk Reduction in Children and Adolescents, released online November 15th, 2011.[28] The recommendations were endorsed by the AAP, and a summary was published in *Pediatrics* on December 1, 2012. For the first time, these guidelines recommend universal screening for lipid disorders. This screening is recommended once between ages 9 and 11 years and again between ages 17 and 21 years. Selective screening continues to be recommended in children aged greater than or equal to 2 years with increased risk, defined as:

- Family history of early atherosclerosis or TC greater than or equal to 240 mg/dL
- High-risk conditions: diabetes, obesity, hypertension, cigarette smoking
- High-risk medical diagnoses: nephrotic syndrome, chronic renal disease, after orthotopic heart transplant, history of Kawasaki disease with persistent coronary involvement, human immunodeficiency virus, chronic inflammatory disease, hypothyroidism
- TC and HDL-C may be obtained to calculate non–HDL-C (TC−HDL-C) or a fasting lipid profile may be obtained for general screening.

There are no prospective studies evaluating the impact of pediatric cholesterol screening on atherosclerotic events, atherosclerosis by autopsy or preclinical vascular testing, or on pediatric or adult cholesterol values per se. There are some reports of the rates of screening using various criteria, and the ability of screening to detect abnormal LDL-C or TC. Based on family history alone, studies suggest that between 20% and 50% of children would be screened for lipid disorders, depending on the population and the methods used for ascertaining family history.[27,29] In Otsego County (NY), 27% of children would have been eligible for screening based on family history of early atherosclerosis and 11% based on family history of hyperlipidemia (total 38%).[30] In a subspecialty clinic, applying major indicators (family history of CVD and lipid disorders) and discretionary indicators (diabetes and hypertension, among others) would have identified 96% of patients with high LDL-C; however, this finding reflects referral bias.[31] In a population of African American children, 37% had NCEP indications for screening[32]; however, this screening strategy would have identified less than 50% of children with LDL-C greater than 130 mg/dL. Similar concerns have been raised for Hispanic children.[33] These studies show that selective screening does not identify most at-risk children.

## LIPID TESTS IN CHILDREN

Various tests have been used for pediatric lipid screening, with variable success. TC levels were originally recommended as screening tests. In the Lipid Research Clinics Study and in NHANES data, the specificity of TC greater than the 95th percentile is reasonable (90%–98%) but the sensitivity is low (50%–69%) to identify LDL-C increases.[2,34] The NHLBI Integrated Guidelines, and also the 2008 AAP Cholesterol Statement, recommend a fasting lipid profile for selective lipid screening; it can also be used for universal screening.[27] Non–HDL-C can now be used as an alternate test for universal screening, a new development that may increase participation in screening. Non-HDL-C, calculated by subtracting HDL-C from TC in a nonfasting sample, is increasingly used in adults, and may better reflect persistently abnormal lipids in children and adolescents, and predict future subclinical atherosclerosis in young adults.[35–37]

For treating lipid disorders, the fasting lipid remains the mainstay of testing in children and adolescents. Assays that directly measure LDL-C are available in most laboratories. These methods are mainly useful in patients who have fasting TGs greater than 400 mg/dL, when the usual method for calculating LDL-C is using the Friedewald calculation. However, direct LDL-C methods either overestimate or underestimate LDL-C (depending on the specific assay) compared with ultracentrifugation, the gold standard research method, and also compared with calculated LDL-C.[38,39] Most practitioners, and all guidelines, do not recommend using direct LDL-C for lipid screening or treatment, except in significant hypertriglyceridemia.

More advanced lipid testing is entering adult clinical practice, although they are not standard.[40] The clinical relevance of advanced lipid testing in children and adolescents is not established, and even normal values are not well defined. However, some information is available from the Bogalusa Cohort on particle size and correlates with cardiovascular risk factor phenotype.[41,42] Apolipoproteins have also been evaluated in Bogalusa, looking specifically at tracking. Apolipoprotein A tracked similarly to HDL-C, whereas apolipoprotein B (apoB) tracked slightly better than LDL-C over time.[43] One study tested the relationship between apolipoproteins and preclinical atherosclerosis. In the Young Finns Study, apoB levels predicted carotid IMT.[44] Advanced lipid testing is not generally used in children, but is likely to become more important over time as understanding of these parameters increases.

## CLINICAL PRESENTATIONS OF LIPID DISORDERS IN CHILDHOOD

A full review of all pediatric lipid disorders is beyond the scope of this article, and these have been reviewed comprehensively elsewhere.[45] This article focuses on 3 main clinical presentations: (1) increased LDL-C and FH, (2) hypertriglyceridemia, and (3) low HDL-C.

### Familial Hyperlipidemias

Past and present pediatric lipid guidelines are primarily directed at detecting and treating FH. The underlying cause of FH is usually 1 of ~1200 described mutations in the gene coding for the LDL-C receptor. A mutation in apoB, the ligand for this receptor, or a cofactor, presents with a similar phenotype. The major features of FH are extremely high LDL-C, and a family history of early atherosclerosis and high cholesterol. HDL-C can also be low in patients with FH but TG levels are normal. FH is common, with a prevalence of 1 in 300 to 500 for the heterozygous form, depending on the population.[46] The heterozygous form of FH is also associated with atherosclerotic events that present during early adulthood, including myocardial infarction, need for coronary revascularization or intervention, peripheral arterial disease, stroke, and renal artery stenosis; 50% of affected men and 25% of affected women have CVD events by the age of 50 years.[47,48] In its homozygous form, FH is associated with rapidly progressive atherosclerosis and cardiovascular events, and frequently mortality from the same conditions, as early as age 2 years, but more commonly in the first and second decade of life.[49] As reviewed later, there are tolerable and safe approaches to reducing LDL-C that presumably modify atherosclerotic risk, including lifestyle improvement, medication, and reducing/preventing other risk factors for CVD, such as obesity, diabetes, hypertension, and cigarette smoking.[14,50–53] Diagnosing a child with FH may help identify other affected adult family members at more immediate risk of CVD.[54]

### Hypertriglyceridemia

Children also present with increased fasting TG levels. Mildly to moderately increased TGs (130–500 mg/dL) are often seen in the context of overweight or obesity, although many overweight children are metabolically preserved or have only mildly abnormal lipid profiles. Patients with these types of profiles may have an increased risk of atherosclerotic events, but often have concurrent CVD risk factors including excess adiposity, insulin resistance, hypertension, poor diet, and inactivity that complicate defining the contribution of high TG levels to CVD risk. Extremely high fasting TG levels (>1000 mg/dL) may be related to uncontrolled diabetes combined with a partial defect in lipoprotein lipase function, complete deficiency/dysfunction of lipoprotein lipase, apolipoprotein C-II deficiency, or other, even rarer conditions.[55] The primary complication of severe hypertriglyceridemia is pancreatitis, which can be life threatening.

### Low HDL-C

Hypoalphalipoproteinemia (low HDL-C) may present as an isolated lipid abnormality, or in concert with high TG or high LDL-C. HDL-C is an important determinant of CVD risk factor in adults. Its role in the pediatric context is not well described, although presumably it is similar to that in adults. Autopsy studies have shown a correlation between low HDL-C levels and the extent of atherosclerosis.[6,9] Obesity, inactivity, and poor intake of healthy fats seem to be important determinants of low HDL-C, although it often runs in families.

Secondary causes of hyperlipidemia should be considered in the pediatric patient. Certain medications are known to increase lipid levels and specific medical disorders can be responsible for a secondary hyperlipidemia. These conditions can usually be excluded by a comprehensive history and physical examination; rarely additional testing is required. It is our current practice to obtain a thyroid-stimulating hormone levels at the time of the first visit to exclude hypothyroidism, a more common correctable reason for hyperlipidemia, and to screen for some additional CVD risk factors (smoking, hypertension, obesity, obesity-related complications including diabetes mellitus). Other evaluations are driven by clinical circumstances.

## LIFESTYLE MODIFICATION OF PEDIATRIC LIPID DISORDERS

The primary management of most pediatric lipid disorders is lifestyle modification. The goals of these interventions are to identify and foster appropriate dietary change, optimize physical activity, limit inactivity, and achieve weight loss if indicated. Exercise has long been recommended to improve all facets of the lipid profile. The data supporting these recommendations in pediatrics is not extensive but improvements have been seen, particularly in TG levels.[56,57]

National guidelines for the nutritional management of all lipid disorders have customarily been uniform, regardless of the specific lipid abnormality. Thus lifestyle modification recommendations have focused on limiting dietary cholesterol, saturated fats, and trans fats. These approaches have been shown to be safe, and somewhat effective in lowering LDL-C. The Dietary Intervention Study in Children (DISC) provided dietary counseling on following a diet low in saturated fats to lower LDL-C levels.[58] Growth and development in the study participants was normal and TC and LDL-C declined slightly.[59] A study of Finnish infants, the Special Turku Coronary Risk Factor Intervention Project (STRIP), showed the safety of dietary counseling for parents on feeding their infants a diet lower in saturated and total fats (goal 30%–35% of dietary intake as fats, one-third as saturated fat). At ~1 year of age, the intervention group had lower TC and LDL-C, without any differences or deficits in growth and development. Differences in dietary intake persisted into early adolescence, with differences in cholesterol seen in boys, and no adverse effects on growth, development, or nutrition.[60]

Dietary interventions to address high TG levels have generally followed closely on the counseling strategies for high LDL-C. However, more recently, focused counseling approaches based on adult data,[61] which are designed to limit total carbohydrate intake and often to affect carbohydrate quality, have been trialed, with some success.[62–64] The 2011 NHLBI Integrated Guidelines for the first time recommend different dietary strategies based on whether LDL-C or TGs are the dominant abnormality. It is also our practice to tailor nutritional advice closely to the specific lipid disorder in the patient.

### Potential Adverse Effects of Lifestyle Modification

Pediatric providers have been concerned about complications related to nutritional treatment of lipid disorders, including excessive weight loss, or failure to gain weight, in children placed on a low-fat diet. Some care must be taken in children who are of normal weight to monitor growth. Anorexia nervosa is the theoretic severe manifestation of this. However, the existing data show that dietary counseling for abnormal lipids is generally safe.[65] Complications of recommendations to increase physical activity include injury in children unused to such exercise, a problem that may be accentuated in overweight children and adolescents. Physical therapy consultation may be useful in severely inactive and/or obese individuals. A gradual start is required. Behavioral disruptions may arise when parents and children address ingrained and emotionally loaded eating practices.

## PHARMACOTHERAPY FOR PEDIATRIC LIPID DISORDERS

Pharmacotherapy is rarely recommended for lipid level modification in children with dyslipidemia. The recent analysis of NHANES data estimated that, despite the presence of some lipid abnormality in one-fifth of the adolescent population, only 1% of children with lipid abnormalities would have met 2008 AAP recommendations for pharmacotherapy.[66] The prevalence of statin therapy in children commercially insured in the United States aged 6 to 18 years between April and June of 2007 was 0.1 per 1000 persons.[67] In clinical practice, lipid-lowering medications are reserved for children with extremely increased LDL-C or TG levels, as described by the NHLBI guidelines.

- The NHLBI Integrated Guidelines recommend pharmacologic treatment when LDL-C is greater than or equal to 190 mg/dL despite 6 or more months of lifestyle modification in patients aged 10 years and older in the absence of additional cardiovascular risk factors or family history of early atherosclerotic disease
- Lower treatment cut-points are advised for children with a family history of early atherosclerosis, or other risk factors (LDL-C $\geq$160 mg/dL).

Risk factors include not only modifiable acquired risk but also medical conditions associated with accelerated atherosclerosis, such as diabetes, chronic renal disease or inflammatory conditions, and heart transplant. The risks associated with these conditions are not well quantified, making the recommendations on exact cut-points a matter of expert opinion.

Statins (3-hydroxy-3-methylglutaryl coenzyme A reductase inhibitors) are first-line pharmacotherapy for LDL-C lowering in children and adolescents, just as they are in adults. Based on ~10 randomized placebo-controlled trials of LDL-C lowering, enrolling primarily children with FH, statins effectively lower LDL-C by 30% to 50%.[68,69] The duration of the trials ranged between 2 months and ~2 years, with 1 trial extended with nonblinded therapy, and encompassed ~1000 patients. Our confidence that rare, subtle, or longer latency side effects can be detected is not high because of the small sample size. Reported complications of statins in children include transaminitis, muscle pain, headache, and nonspecific gastrointestinal side effects; rhabdomyolysis has not been reported in children or adolescents. A few of our patients have notified us of psychiatric symptoms associated with the use of statins, such as irritability, depression, and mood changes; this is anecdotal experience.

There is a growing appreciation of an association between statin therapy and a small increase in the risk of diabetes mellitus type 2. A meta-analysis of 13 large randomized controlled trials of statin use in adults showed a 9% increased incidence of diabetes mellitus over the course of 4 years.[70] This effect may be mediated through insulin resistance, although obesity did not emerge as a contributor to this phenomenon in the meta-analysis of adult statin trials. There are no data currently available on this topic in children or adolescents.

Other lipid-lowering therapies have been used in childhood, including fenofibrates,[71] ezetimibe, bile acid binding resins, niacin[72] and derivatives, and neutraceuticals such as stanol esters and ω-3 fatty acid supplements. Stanols effectively lower LDL-C in children by ~10%, but their use has not been shown to lower rates of CVD in adults. The available literature on fibrates is sparse,[71] but they have been used to try to reduce the risk of pancreatitis in patients with significant TG increases who have insulin resistance as part of their clinical picture. Whether this is effective in children or adolescents is untested.

### Cardiovascular Testing

No cardiology testing is required for the routine pediatric patient with abnormal lipids, aside from the rare individual with homozygous FH. Noninvasive vascular testing has been used in research protocols as an outcome measure, but is not generally available clinically. The armamentarium for assessing atherosclerosis in research has expanded to include peripheral testing of proximal vessel function (brachial artery reactivity testing), distal vessel function (endoPAT), vascular stiffness (using arterial tonometry), and vessel thickening (carotid IMT). Each of these tests seems to give information about a different aspect of vascular health. There are several reports of improvement in these vascular tests with therapies that reduce cardiovascular risk (discussed earlier). However, the connection between abnormal testing during childhood and adult disease events has not been made convincingly, and these tests are not used clinically.

### CONTROVERSY ABOUT PEDIATRIC LIPID SCREENING AND TREATMENT

Pediatric cholesterol screening is extremely controversial.[32,73–76] In 2007, the United States Preventive Services Task Force (USPSTF) systematically reviewed the evidence to answer select questions on topics related to childhood lipid screening and treatment.[29,77] Despite generally being in agreement about the link between childhood and adult lipid disorders, the usefulness of some lipid testing to detect childhood lipid disorders, and the effectiveness of statin medications in reducing LDL-C in FH, they noted the lack of available randomized controlled trials connecting pediatric screening and changes in childhood lipid levels to improved adult health outcomes, and the evidence was insufficient to support a recommendation either for or against screening or treating pediatric lipid disorders.[29] The Task Force was composed of providers outside pediatric preventive cardiology, and mostly nonpediatricians. In the absence of sufficient data, they gave no clinical guidelines for screening or management.

The recent NHLBI recommendation for universal screening is more aggressive about lipid management in children, with its recommendation for universal screening twice during childhood and adolescence in addition to selective screening. It is unclear how universal screening will affect the identification rates. Although the numbers of children with abnormal lipids is likely to increase, the detection of severe lipid disorders may not increase change greatly, because the pool tested by selective screening is expected to be at higher pretest probability. The impact of pediatric cholesterol screening has not been prospective evaluated. Compliance with lipid screening on the part of the patient and family has been poor in the past[32]; none of the available literature assesses the patient experience of lipid screening. Furthermore, it is unclear how well cholesterol screening guidelines have been adopted by pediatric providers. Adoption of screening and treatment guidelines by providers is not universal. These recommendations may impose a substantial burden on the health care system and are untested for identification rates, cost, burden on providers and families, and efficacy in modifying lipid abnormalities.

Reaction to pediatric lipid guidelines is heated.[78-80] Some of the strength of the reaction may be fear about inappropriate prescribing of lipid-lowering medications to children and adolescents who could fix their cholesterol problems by eating better, exercising more, and losing weight. More comprehensive lifestyle change supports are often suggested by those who argue against pediatric statin therapy. No one treating these children would object to more comprehensive medical, social, and (most importantly) environmental supports to following a heart-healthy lifestyle. Most children and adolescents who meet pharmacologic criteria for high LDL-C are likely to have genetic contributors, and, with rare exceptions, everyone who gets pharmacotherapy should have greater than or equal to 6 months of lifestyle change before medications are initiated. The evidence base for pediatric lipid screening and management is not complete, but, in the absence of perfection, action is still required.

## LITERATURE GAPS

There are important gaps in the literature on the effect of pediatric lipid screening and treatment on lipid lowering and CVD event reduction. Rigorous randomized trial designs using CVD events as outcomes are unlikely to be accomplished, partly because of the 30-year to 50-year latency between exposure and events. However, avenues exist for improving understanding and practice around pediatric lipid disorders:

- Expand the use of novel outcomes in research to include new or more established preclinical vascular testing
- Go beyond prevention of CVD events, and aim to prevent or modify the risk factor (primordial prevention)
- Improve understanding of provider, parental, and patient attitudes and behavior around lipid abnormalities to better understand adoption rates and determinants (characteristics of providers, patients, family, and systems)
- Cost-effectiveness analysis of pediatric lipid screening
- Form registries of children on long-term statin therapy, starting in childhood
- Evaluate the role of advanced lipid testing in pediatrics
- Determine the clinical usefulness of genetic testing, specifically determine whether genetic diagnoses affect response to therapy, screening method, or clinical outcomes in FH
- Determine whether statins should be used in the adolescent with NAFLD

- Determine whether the choice of lipid-lowering therapy should be modified according to the risk of diabetes reported in adult trial data.

## SUMMARY

Improving childhood cholesterol lipid disorders is an important public health issue. The approach of targeting childhood lipid disorders to address CVD reduction during adulthood is recommended because of the data connecting childhood lipid disorders to atherosclerosis. Although definitive proof that reduction of childhood lipid concentrations decreases CVD later in life is not yet available, supporting evidence continues to accrue. Identifying and modifying lipid disorders during childhood may modify the outcome of distant clinical atherosclerotic disease. However, this question should be examined as rigorously and as creatively as possible. While the evidence base continues to grow, the most prudent approach for pediatric providers may be to follow NHLBI Integrated Guidelines while actively pursuing research that will close gaps in the literature on this topic.[27]

## REFERENCES

1. Prevalence of abnormal lipid levels among youths – United States, 1999-2006. MMWR Morb Mortal Wkly Rep 2010;59(2):29–33.
2. Hickman TB, Briefel RR, Carroll MD, et al. Distributions and trends of serum lipid levels among United States children and adolescents ages 4-19 years: data from the Third National Health and Nutrition Examination Survey. Prev Med 1998;27(6): 879–90.
3. Winkleby MA, Robinson TN, Sundquist J, et al. Ethnic variation in cardiovascular disease risk factors among children and young adults: findings from the Third National Health and Nutrition Examination Survey, 1988-1994. JAMA 1999; 281(11):1006–13.
4. Roger VL, Go AS, Lloyd-Jones DM, et al. Heart disease and stroke statistics–2011 update: a report from the American Heart Association. Circulation 2011; 123(4):e18–209.
5. Stary HC. Evolution and progression of atherosclerotic lesions in coronary arteries of children and young adults. Arteriosclerosis 1989;9(Suppl 1):I19–32.
6. McGill HC Jr, McMahan CA. Determinants of atherosclerosis in the young. Pathobiological Determinants of Atherosclerosis in Youth (PDAY) Research Group. Am J Cardiol 1998;82(10B):30T–6T.
7. Franks PW, Hanson RL, Knowler WC, et al. Childhood obesity, other cardiovascular risk factors, and premature death. N Engl J Med 2010;362(6):485–93.
8. Morrison JA, Glueck CJ, Wang P. Childhood risk factors predict cardiovascular disease, impaired fasting glucose plus type 2 diabetes mellitus, and high blood pressure 26 years later at a mean age of 38 years: the Princeton-lipid research clinics follow-up study. Metabolism 2011. [Epub ahead of print].
9. Newman WP III, Freedman DS, Voors AW, et al. Relation of serum lipoprotein levels and systolic blood pressure to early atherosclerosis. The Bogalusa Heart Study. N Engl J Med 1986;314(3):138–44.
10. Berenson GS, Srinivasan SR, Bao W, et al. Association between multiple cardiovascular risk factors and atherosclerosis in children and young adults. The Bogalusa Heart Study. N Engl J Med 1998;338(23):1650–6.
11. Davis PH, Dawson JD, Riley WA, et al. Carotid intimal-medial thickness is related to cardiovascular risk factors measured from childhood through middle age: the Muscatine Study. Circulation 2001;104(23):2815–9.

12. Davis PH, Dawson JD, Mahoney LT, et al. Increased carotid intimal-medial thickness and coronary calcification are related in young and middle-aged adults. The Muscatine Study. Circulation 1999;100(8):838–42.

13. Paul TK, Srinivasan SR, Wei C, et al. Cardiovascular risk profile of asymptomatic healthy young adults with increased femoral artery intima-media thickness: the Bogalusa Heart Study. Am J Med Sci 2005;330(3):105–10.

14. Wiegman A, Hutten BA, de Groot E, et al. Efficacy and safety of statin therapy in children with familial hypercholesterolemia: a randomized controlled trial. JAMA 2004;292(3):331–7.

15. Rodenburg J, Vissers MN, Wiegman A, et al. Statin treatment in children with familial hypercholesterolemia: the younger, the better. Circulation 2007;116(6): 664–8.

16. Austin MA, Hutter CM, Zimmern RL, et al. Genetic causes of monogenic heterozygous familial hypercholesterolemia: a HuGE prevalence review. Am J Epidemiol 2004;160(5):407–20.

17. Cohen JC, Boerwinkle E, Mosley TH Jr, et al. Sequence variations in PCSK9, low LDL, and protection against coronary heart disease. N Engl J Med 2006;354(12): 1264–72.

18. Clarke WR, Schrott HG, Leaverton PE, et al. Tracking of blood lipids and blood pressures in school age children: the Muscatine Study. Circulation 1978;58(4): 626–34.

19. Stuhldreher W, Donahue R, Drash A, et al. The Beaver County Lipid Study. Sixteen-year cholesterol tracking. Ann N Y Acad Sci 1991;623:466–8.

20. Juhola J, Magnussen CG, Viikari JS, et al. Tracking of serum lipid levels, blood pressure, and body mass index from childhood to adulthood: the Cardiovascular Risk in Young Finns Study. J Pediatr 2011;159(4):584–90.

21. Webber LS, Srinivasan SR, Wattigney WA, et al. Tracking of serum lipids and lipoproteins from childhood to adulthood. The Bogalusa Heart Study. Am J Epidemiol 1991;133(9):884–99.

22. Gillman MW. Screening for familial hypercholesterolemia in childhood. Am J Dis Child 1993;147(4):393–6.

23. American Academy of Pediatrics Committee on Nutrition: prudent life-style for children: dietary fat and cholesterol. Pediatrics 1986;78(3):521–5.

24. National Cholesterol Education Program (NCEP): highlights of the report of the Expert Panel on Blood Cholesterol Levels in Children and Adolescents. Pediatrics 1992;89(3):495–501.

25. American Academy of Pediatrics Committee on Nutrition: statement on cholesterol. Pediatrics 1992;90(3):469–73.

26. American Academy of Pediatrics. Committee on nutrition. Cholesterol in childhood. Pediatrics 1998;101(1 Pt 1):141–7.

27. Daniels SR, Greer FR. Lipid screening and cardiovascular health in childhood. Pediatrics 2008;122(1):198–208.

28. Expert panel on integrated guidelines for cardiovascular health and risk reduction in children and adolescents: summary report. Pediatrics 2011;128(Suppl 5): S213–56.

29. Haney EM, Huffman LH, Bougatsos C, et al. Screening and treatment for lipid disorders in children and adolescents: systematic evidence review for the US Preventive Services Task Force. Pediatrics 2007;120(1):e189–214.

30. Dennison BA, Jenkins PL, Pearson TA. Challenges to implementing the current pediatric cholesterol screening guidelines into practice. Pediatrics 1994;94(3): 296–302.

31. Diller PM, Huster GA, Leach AD, et al. Definition and application of the discretionary screening indicators according to the National Cholesterol Education Program for Children and Adolescents. J Pediatr 1995;126(3):345–52.
32. Rifai N, Neufeld E, Ahlstrom P, et al. Failure of current guidelines for cholesterol screening in urban African-American adolescents. Pediatrics 1996;98(3 Pt 1): 383–8.
33. Shea S, Basch CE, Irigoyen M, et al. Failure of family history to predict high blood cholesterol among Hispanic preschool children. Prev Med 1990;19(4):443–55.
34. LaRosa JC, Chambless LE, Criqui MH, et al. Patterns of dyslipoproteinemia in selected North American populations. The Lipid Research Clinics Program Prevalence Study. Circulation 1986;73(1 Pt 2):I12–29.
35. Kastelein JJ, van der Steeg WA, Holme I, et al. Lipids, apolipoproteins, and their ratios in relation to cardiovascular events with statin treatment. Circulation 2008; 117(23):3002–9.
36. Frontini MG, Srinivasan SR, Xu JH, et al. Utility of non-high-density lipoprotein cholesterol versus other lipoprotein measures in detecting subclinical atherosclerosis in young adults (the Bogalusa Heart Study). Am J Cardiol 2007;100(1):64–8.
37. Srinivasan SR, Frontini MG, Xu J, et al. Utility of childhood non-high-density lipoprotein cholesterol levels in predicting adult dyslipidemia and other cardiovascular risks: the Bogalusa Heart Study. Pediatrics 2006;118(1):201–6.
38. Yu HH, Markowitz R, de Ferranti SD, et al. Direct measurement of LDL-C in children: performance of two surfactant-based methods in a general pediatric population. Clin Biochem 2000;33(2):89–95.
39. de Ferranti S, Shapiro D, Markowitz R, et al. Nonfasting low-density lipoprotein testing: utility for cholesterol screening in pediatric primary care. Clin Pediatr (Phila) 2007;46(5):441–5.
40. Davidson MH, Ballantyne CM, Jacobson TA, et al. Clinical utility of inflammatory markers and advanced lipoprotein testing: advice from an expert panel of lipid specialists. J Clin Lipidol 2011;5(5):338–67.
41. Freedman DS, Bowman BA, Otvos JD, et al. Levels and correlates of LDL and VLDL particle sizes among children: the Bogalusa Heart Study. Atherosclerosis 2000;152(2):441–9.
42. Freedman DS, Bowman BA, Srinivasan SR, et al. Distribution and correlates of high-density lipoprotein subclasses among children and adolescents. Metabolism 2001;50(3):370–6.
43. Bao W, Srinivasan SR, Berenson GS. Tracking of serum apolipoproteins A-I and B in children and young adults: the Bogalusa Heart Study. J Clin Epidemiol 1993; 46(7):609–16.
44. Mattsson N, Magnussen CG, Ronnemaa T, et al. Metabolic syndrome and carotid intima-media thickness in young adults: roles of apolipoprotein B, apolipoprotein A-I, C-reactive protein, and secretory phospholipase A2. The Cardiovascular Risk in Young Finns Study. Arterioscler Thromb Vasc Biol 2010;30(9):1861–6. [Epub 2010 Jun 10].
45. Available at: http://www.nhlbi.nih.gov/guidelines/cvd_ped/chapter9.htm#_ednref16. Accessed January 22, 2012.
46. Hopkins PN, Toth PP, Ballantyne CM, et al. Familial hypercholesterolemias: prevalence, genetics, diagnosis and screening recommendations from the National Lipid Association Expert Panel on Familial Hypercholesterolemia. J Clin Lipidol 2011;5(Suppl 3):S9–17.
47. Marks D, Thorogood M, Neil HA, et al. A review on the diagnosis, natural history, and treatment of familial hypercholesterolaemia. Atherosclerosis 2003;168(1):1–14.

48. Hazzard WR, Goldstein JL, Schrott MG, et al. Hyperlipidemia in coronary heart disease. 3. Evaluation of lipoprotein phenotypes of 156 genetically defined survivors of myocardial infarction. J Clin Invest 1973;52(7):1569–77.
49. Allen JM, Thompson GR, Myant NB, et al. Cardiovascular complications of homozygous familial hypercholesterolaemia. Br Heart J 1980;44(4):361–8.
50. Kavey RE, Daniels SR, Lauer RM, et al. American Heart Association guidelines for primary prevention of atherosclerotic cardiovascular disease beginning in childhood. J Pediatr 2003;142(4):368–72.
51. Obarzanek E, Kimm SY, Barton BA, et al. Long-term safety and efficacy of a cholesterol-lowering diet in children with elevated low-density lipoprotein cholesterol: seven-year results of the Dietary Intervention Study in Children (DISC). Pediatrics 2001;107(2):256–64.
52. Daniels SR, Gidding SS, de Ferranti SD. Pediatric aspects of familial hypercholesterolemias: recommendations from the National Lipid Association Expert Panel on Familial Hypercholesterolemia. J Clin Lipidol 2011;5(Suppl 3):S30–7.
53. Kavey RE, Allada V, Daniels SR, et al. Cardiovascular risk reduction in high-risk pediatric patients: a scientific statement from the American Heart Association Expert Panel on Population and Prevention Science; the Councils on Cardiovascular Disease in the Young, Epidemiology and Prevention, Nutrition, Physical Activity and Metabolism, High Blood Pressure Research, Cardiovascular Nursing, and the Kidney in Heart Disease; and the Interdisciplinary Working Group on Quality of Care and Outcomes Research: endorsed by the American Academy of Pediatrics. Circulation 2006;114(24):2710–38.
54. Marks D, Wonderling D, Thorogood M, et al. Screening for hypercholesterolaemia versus case finding for familial hypercholesterolaemia: a systematic review and cost-effectiveness analysis. Health Technol Assess 2000;4(29):1–123.
55. Kwiterovich PO Jr. Recognition and management of dyslipidemia in children and adolescents. J Clin Endocrinol Metab 2008;93(11):4200–9.
56. Ferguson MA, Gutin B, Le NA, et al. Effects of exercise training and its cessation on components of the insulin resistance syndrome in obese children. Int J Obes Relat Metab Disord 1999;23(8):889–95.
57. Ebbeling CB, Rodriguez NR. Effects of exercise combined with diet therapy on protein utilization in obese children. Med Sci Sports Exerc 1999;31(3):378–85.
58. Lauer RM, Obarzanek E, Hunsberger SA, et al. Efficacy and safety of lowering dietary intake of total fat, saturated fat, and cholesterol in children with elevated LDL cholesterol: the Dietary Intervention Study in Children. Am J Clin Nutr 2000;72(Suppl 5):1332S–42S.
59. Kwiterovich PO Jr, Barton BA, McMahon RP, et al. Effects of diet and sexual maturation on low-density lipoprotein cholesterol during puberty: the Dietary Intervention Study in Children (DISC). Circulation 1997;96(8):2526–33.
60. Niinikoski H, Lagstrom H, Jokinen E, et al. Impact of repeated dietary counseling between infancy and 14 years of age on dietary intakes and serum lipids and lipoproteins. The STRIP Study. Circulation 2007;116(9):1032–40.
61. Pieke B, von EA, Gulbahce E, et al. Treatment of hypertriglyceridemia by two diets rich either in unsaturated fatty acids or in carbohydrates: effects on lipoprotein subclasses, lipolytic enzymes, lipid transfer proteins, insulin and leptin. Int J Obes Relat Metab Disord 2000;24(10):1286–96.
62. Ohta T, Nakamura R, Ikeda Y, et al. Follow up study on children with dyslipidaemia detected by mass screening at 18 months of age: effect of 12 months dietary treatment. Eur J Pediatr 1993;152(11):939–43.

63. Ebbeling CB, Leidig MM, Sinclair KB, et al. A reduced-glycemic load diet in the treatment of adolescent obesity. Arch Pediatr Adolesc Med 2003;157(8):773–9.
64. Ebbeling CB, Leidig MM, Feldman HA, et al. Effects of a low-glycemic load vs low-fat diet in obese young adults: a randomized trial. JAMA 2007;297(19):2092–102.
65. Clauss SB, Kwiterovich PO. Long-term safety and efficacy of low-fat diets in children and adolescents. Minerva Pediatr 2002;54(4):305–13.
66. Centers for Disease Control and Prevention (CDC). Prevalence of abnormal lipid levels among youths – United States, 1999-2006. MMWR Morb Mortal Wkly Rep 2010;59(2):29–33.
67. Liberman JN, Berger JE, Lewis M. Prevalence of antihypertensive, antidiabetic, and dyslipidemic prescription medication use among children and adolescents. Arch Pediatr Adolesc Med 2009;163(4):357–64.
68. Gandelman K, Glue P, Laskey R, et al. An eight-week trial investigating the efficacy and tolerability of atorvastatin for children and adolescents with heterozygous familial hypercholesterolemia. Pediatr Cardiol 2011;32(4):433–41.
69. Avis HJ, Hutten BA, Gagne C, et al. Efficacy and safety of rosuvastatin therapy for children with familial hypercholesterolemia. J Am Coll Cardiol 2010;55(11):1121–6.
70. Sattar N, Preiss D, Murray HM, et al. Statins and risk of incident diabetes: a collaborative meta-analysis of randomised statin trials. Lancet 2010;375(9716):735–42.
71. Wheeler KA, West RJ, Lloyd JK, et al. Double blind trial of bezafibrate in familial hypercholesterolaemia. Arch Dis Child 1985;60(1):34–7.
72. Colletti RB, Neufeld EJ, Roff NK, et al. Niacin treatment of hypercholesterolemia in children. Pediatrics 1993;92(1):78–82.
73. Szamosi T, Keltai M, Romics L, et al. Screening of children with high familial risk of arteriosclerosis. Acta Paediatr Hung 1985;26(3):187–91.
74. O'Loughlin J, Lauzon B, Paradis G, et al. Usefulness of the American Academy of Pediatrics recommendations for identifying youths with hypercholesterolemia. Pediatrics 2004;113(6):1723–7.
75. Merz B. New studies fuel controversy over universal cholesterol screening during childhood. JAMA 1989;261(6):814.
76. Kuehl KS. Cholesterol screening in childhood. Targeted versus universal approaches. Ann N Y Acad Sci 1991;623:193–9.
77. Grossman DC, Moyer VA, Melnyk BM, et al. The anatomy of a US Preventive Services Task Force recommendation: lipid screening for children and adolescents. Arch Pediatr Adolesc Med 2011;165(3):205–10.
78. Gillman MW, Daniels SR. Is universal pediatric lipid screening justified? JAMA 2012;307(3):259–60.
79. Psaty BM, Rivara FP. Universal screening and drug treatment of dyslipidemia in children and adolescents. JAMA 2012;307(3):257–8.
80. de Ferranti S, Ludwig DS. Storm over statins–the controversy surrounding pharmacologic treatment of children. N Engl J Med 2008;359(13):1309–12.

# Index

*Note:* Page numbers of article titles are in **boldface** type.

## A

Med Clin N Am 96 (2012) 155–164
doi:10.1016/S0025-7125(12)00036-3
0025-7125/12/$ – see front matter © 2012 Elsevier Inc. All rights reserved.

medical.theclinics.com

# Moving?

## Make sure your subscription moves with you!

To notify us of your new address, find your **Clinics Account Number** (located on your mailing label above your name), and contact customer service at:

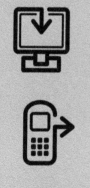

**Email: journalscustomerservice-usa@elsevier.com**

**800-654-2452** (subscribers in the U.S. & Canada)
**314-447-8871** (subscribers outside of the U.S. & Canada)

**Fax number: 314-447-8029**

**Elsevier Health Sciences Division**
**Subscription Customer Service**
**3251 Riverport Lane**
**Maryland Heights, MO 63043**

*To ensure uninterrupted delivery of your subscription, please notify us at least 4 weeks in advance of move.

Printed and bound by CPI Group (UK) Ltd, Croydon, CR0 4YY

08/06/2025

01896875-0009